OUT OF THE DARKNESS

Kate Simonet

Acknowledgments

For my parents and my sister, Ann. Without your unconditional love and never-ending support, I would not be alive or where I am today.

For my best friend, Kylie. Thank you for over twenty years of friendship and staying by my side in my darkest times.

For my therapist, Richard. You have helped me face the most beautiful and ugly parts of my life. It has been difficult but extremely eye opening. Most of all, you have helped me to find freedom and peace.

For Ricky. Thank you for loving me for who I truly am and accepting all of me. You bring out the best in me. I love you with all of my heart.

For Grandpa. Thank you for teaching me that happiness is a choice and for helping me be a better version of myself without even knowing it.

For everyone who struggles with mental health issues. I hope this book gives you hope and lets you know you are not alone.

Disclaimer:

This book is a memoir. The contents of this book are for informational purposes only. The content is not intended to be a substitute for professional advice, diagnosis, or treatment. Always seek the advice of your mental health professional or other qualified health provider with any questions you may have regarding your condition. Never disregard professional advice or delay in seeking it because of something you have read in this book.

The story contains content that might be troubling for some readers including, but not limited to, depictions and references regarding death, suicide, and vivid nightmare imagery. Please be mindful of these as possible triggers and seek support if needed.

I have tried to recreate events, locations and conversations from my memory. In order to maintain anonymity in some instances I have changed the names of individuals and places.

Contents

Introduction

As a senior in high school, I had what many would call an "All-American Life." I was varsity captain in three sports, was named the most athletic female in my highschool, an academic honors student, and, in seven short months, I would be on my way to a Division II college to pursue my education and compete on the cross country and track team. My parents are supportive and married. I have a loving sister. I was truly happy and thankful for the life I had and all the hard work I had put in to get me to where I was.

Despite this "All-American" background, nothing had prepared me for the downward spiral that led me to two, two-weeklong psychiatric hospitalization stays and a suicide attempt before those seven months were up. I would later be diagnosed with Bipolar Disorder and, with time, learn to overcome stigma, and eventually find peace and learn to live a successful and meaningful life.

If I had a better understanding of what mental illnesses looked like and had the correct resources and language to ask for help, things would not have been so difficult for my younger self. I believe that if my parents and friends had known more about mental health issues I would not have had to go through what I did.

I wish there were more awareness and education of how mental health issues can affect even a successful, driven, loved, and supportive kid. I don't want what happened to me to happen to anyone else. I hope by sharing my story I can bring awareness to mental health and give the reader a sense of hope. If people do not share their experiences, how do we learn from one another and help each other along the way?

"What's broken can be mended. What hurts can be healed. And no matter how dark it gets, the sun is going to rise again."

— Unknown

A Warning Sign

In high school I was known for being athletic. I was a three-sport athlete: cross country in the fall, basketball in the winter, and track in the spring. My junior year was a year to remember when it came to the sport of cross country.

My sister, Ann, and I ran high school cross country together. Ann is four years younger. She's smart, athletic, one of the kindest and hardest-working people I know. Not to mention she takes zero shit from anyone. We are very different. I would describe my sixteen-year-old self as extremely nice, quiet, hard-working, an overthinker, and a perfectionist. The sport brought us closer. It felt special to be in a sport with my sister and to both be talented at it made it feel even more remarkable. We both qualified for the Minnesota State Cross Country Championships this year. Ann was just a seventh grader.

The state final was a race to remember. The local newspaper read: "Simonet Sisters Head to State." We were in the spotlight and toeing the line for the state cross country meet, held in Northfield, MN. I was in prime shape, mentally prepared, and excited to compete. We had friends and family lining the back of the start line holding hand-made signs with little mantras to help cheer us on. I loved seeing all of my favorite people in one spot and it meant so much to me that they made the trip out to the course to watch us race.

With only seven minutes before the starting gun, Ann realized she did not have the timing chips laced to her shoes. In larger cross country meets, the officials use chips which athletes wear on their shoes throughout the race. It gives accurate timing as to when we cross certain mile points and also gives the officials a final time of the race for each runner. Without the chip, Ann's time and place would not count.

Pure panic sunk in. Our teammates and coaches were scrambling to locate Ann's chips. I stopped thinking about my race strategy and became completely focused on Ann. I did my best to stay calm and also keep her calm. The team rummaged through the van we took to get to the course and had no luck. Time was ticking down and, thankfully, our head coach was able to get a replacement set of chips from the race coordinators.

For me, the race did not go as planned. I was mentally checked out due to the events that preceded it and didn't place where I wanted to. As I made my way throughout the course, I was so thrown off by the fact that Ann's time and place almost didn't matter, and was unable to get in my pre-race mindset. Ann and I ran together the first half of the race before she broke away. I felt stressed and distracted throughout the race. The course was lined with people cheering and shaking cowbells, but all of the noise seemed muffled and the bodies seemed blurry.

Even though I did not finish where I wanted to my junior year, it will always be a fond memory. It is one of my favorite memories from high school. Now that we're both older, we talk about that day with a smile on our face and often laugh at the fact that after the race our underwear was spread throughout the van from when our teammates and coaches were searching for Ann's racing chip.

When we arrived back to our hometown, my parents threw us a large surprise party in our family's garage. Friends and family came from all around to celebrate our trip to the state meet. It was a wonderful day and it felt extra special to be surrounded by so many loved ones.

As I reflect on this moment, I wonder why my performance was so impacted by Ann's situation when she seemed to be unaltered. I was always concerned about how others were feeling and worried about their experience to the point that it physically and mentally affected me. Could this have been a warning sign for what was ahead?

A Taste of Depression

It was a Friday in October 2012, just a year after we had qualified for State. I was seventeen, a senior in high school, and the day before I had just finished my last race as a high school cross country runner. It was a disappointing race. I was underprepared and the weather conditions weren't ideal. It was cold and rainy. My clothes were sopping wet from the rain and my legs felt numb as I crossed the finish line. I didn't have it in me to finish in the top ten spots needed to advance to the state meet that would be taking place in November. I walked off the course not quite comprehending that it was all over. My dad met me at the team tent, gave me such a big hug, and I cried into his arms. He reminded me that my running career was far from over.

Qualifying for this race was very important to me as I had been accepted to run on the Division II cross country and track team beginning my freshman year of college. I wanted to end my high school career on a good note before advancing to bigger things.

On the Friday following my last race of senior year, I felt run down, disappointed, and mentally exhausted. I asked my mom if I could take the day off from school to just relax and watch movies. My mom was happy to allow me to stay home from school, and I spent the day watching my favorite series, Harry Potter. The reason I call this day out is because it was a turning point in my life. I didn't know it at the time, but it would be the first time I had ever experienced a hint of depression.

Baby Cakes

Days passed and we were now into basketball season at my high school. This was another sport Ann and I played together; however, we were on separate teams. I wasn't the best at basketball, but it was always a fun time of year because I was able to play and laugh my way through practices with my best friend, Kylie. We were named captains together that season.

Kylie and I go back a long time. We have been friends since first grade and she was, and is, one of the closest and dearest people in my life. Each year we would apply for the same classes, ride to school together when our schedules aligned, go to the local donut shop together after Saturday morning practices, and almost always hang out together on the weekends. She knew me better than anyone else at the time and she made going to school fun and exciting. Kylie is a lot like my sister. She was more outgoing and social than I was and always pushed me out of my comfort zone and made me feel included.

Before practice, at least once a week, you could find us in my parents' kitchen baking a new flavored cupcake. We were well organized with our layout of the kitchen and almost always had the new Taylor Swift CD playing in the background. We would find so much joy planning out each week's cupcake. We exchanged notes back and forth leading up to the baking day, selecting flavors and including design options. We would imagine ourselves opening a bakery when we were older; I would be the main baker and she would do the marketing. Kylie and I would call our start up business Baby Cakes.

If I can recall, our favorite cupcake we ever made was a mocha cupcake; it had coffee mixed within the chocolate cake, espresso, buttercream frosting, and we topped it off with a chocolate covered coffee bean. We often posted pictures to Instagram showing off our work.

As time went by, we invested in nicer baking supplies, colorful and sparkly cupcake liners, and different shapes and sizes of frosting tips. Each time we finished a batch, we would split one of the cupcakes in half and taste it. If we found it as delicious as we hoped, we would bring the batch to the next basketball game to share with our teammates.

During our baking sessions we often sang along to the lyrics from Taylor's CD, laughed, and talked about what we wanted our future husbands to be like. I always imagined someone very athletic, who appreciated the outdoors, and who loved my family's cabin as much as I did. Kylie always spoke of someone tall, dark, and handsome. She also really wanted kids one day, as did I. I wanted that for her. We would always promise each other we'd be at each other's wedding when we did meet our dream boys.

Grasping for Perfection

I was very driven to be in top-notch shape come track season in the spring, so after basketball practices I would go up to the local gym and run on the treadmill. I was focused on qualifying for State for track and didn't want the off-season from running to hinder my endurance. During this time, I began to be more aware of my body image. I didn't compare myself to other young women, but I believed that if I were smaller, I would be able to run more efficiently. I began to cut calories, eat what I thought were "clean" foods, and set certain times in my day that I was only allowed to eat. Anything to get an edge over my competitors. I honestly think that I was so obsessive with my training and eating habits because I needed to be controlling something. I thought if I could take control of my performance, race times, and outward appearance, I could control my mood and happiness. It was very skewed thinking.

I had just had my eighteenth birthday and it was Thanksgiving. Since that day back in October, the initial feeling of exhaustion persisted, accompanied by a sense of anxiety and stress. I brushed it off as being overwhelmed with school work and my busy schedule. We spent Thanksgiving at my aunt and uncle's house in Minneapolis. This was a very special Thanksgiving because most years we did not celebrate with my grandparents and they drove into town on this occasion.

While there, I spent a great deal of time with my grandpa, laughing and telling old stories. He is one of my favorite people, I could listen to that man talk for hours and not get bored. His stories always had a life lesson in them, and I never wanted to miss anything he said. He pulled me aside that day and told me to find joy in my sports and not be too hard on myself. I think he could see how much energy I put into competing. He always wanted me to "just have fun" with what I was doing and I appreciated that. This was not the first or last time my Grandpa gave me this reminder.

Basketball season was well underway. Between my advanced classes, basketball, and running, I had a lot to juggle. The stress persisted. I found myself losing interest in interacting with my friends and classmates. In English class one day, I was sitting back in the classroom away from everyone else. Kylie came back to me and asked if I wanted to come and join the table up front. I took her up on her offer, thinking to myself how exhausting it sounded to have to interact with anyone else.

Generally, you would think being more tired would cause me to oversleep; however, I would often be up most nights, tossing and turning. Some nights I would lay awake just staring at the ceiling, but most nights I would rack my brain trying to solve what was wrong with me. *Why wasn't I happy?* I would ask myself, feeling extremely guilty for feeling this way because I had a good life. There was nothing to complain about. Others had it much worse than I did. How dare I feel this way when my hard work was paying off?

Still, I felt unsatisfied and a sense of hollowness in me. I decided I needed to be a better person. I believed if I worked harder, was nicer, was more popular, and went to church more often, these feelings would cease to exist. So that is what I did.

I became more strict with my running regiment. I began to train before school and sometimes after school as well. I wrote workouts for myself and all of my runs were a minimum of five miles a day. I was restricting and purging my food most days in order to become faster and skinnier. I made a point to go to church every Sunday to talk to God and ask him to make me a better person so I could be happy again.

I made myself go to more social events outside of school to spend time with friends, and I also spent more time studying and doing homework in order to get better grades. I needed to hide these bad feelings I was having because I wanted others to believe I was happy. If I could, I would go back and hug my younger self and tell her she was enough; she just needs to be herself, and it's okay to feel the way she is feeling. I would squeeze her and tell her to open up to her teachers, coaches, family, and friends. I can't go back, but if I could, I would tell my family, coaches, and teachers how I was feeling. I would confidently tell them that I needed help and that I couldn't deal with my symptoms alone. I would not try so hard at being perfect or pleasing others.

Feeling Alone

Our assistant basketball coach, Sellberg, was always fun and seemed to like me. Throughout the season of my senior year, he would often pull me aside and ask how I was doing in school and outside of basketball. I'm not sure if this man had a special sense, but he always seemed a little concerned. At the time, I viewed him as someone who could see through my fake smile, and to me, that was not a good thing. I viewed my sadness and pain as a weakness and terrible flaw. I was ashamed because I thought I was taking my life for granted and that I needed to be "better" and just suck it up. I wish I could go back and tell Sellberg how I was actually doing. As weeks went by, he would pull me aside more often and ask me if he could do anything for me. I would always brush him off with a fake laugh and smile and try to limit my time around him. Throughout my downward spiral into depression, he was the only adult within school or in my sports to mentally check on me and could tell something was very wrong. However, Kylie and some of my other closer friends began to see through things too, but these girls did not have the education or knowledge on mental health issues either. They only thought I didn't want to hang out with them, and I am sure that made them feel bad, though that was not my intent. Because I was withdrawing and being more quiet, I got the sense that this made them question our friendship and hurt their feelings. I didn't know how to tell them that it wasn't them at all. I believed I was a problem and in a way viewed myself as a burden to them.

One night I was at a boys' home basketball game. While sitting in the stands, I felt very alone even though the stands were full. I got up and walked to the bathroom and broke into tears. Overwhelmed with sadness, I was almost surprised by the pain that had arisen within me. It felt good to cry. My friend Kaitlyn happened to walk in and asked if I were all right. I told her I was sad and had no idea why. We were the only ones in the bathroom just outside the gym. You could hear the cheers of the crowd muffled in the background. I felt safe and relieved that she walked in.

Kaitlyn was another close friend in the group with Kylie and I. With her giving and gentle heart, she was there in times I needed consoling. Whether frustrated or excited, Kaitlyn was a good person to share my feelings with. In the bathroom I opened up to her and told her sometimes I just cry, for no reason at all. "I just get really sad," I said. Kaitlyn, being her dear self, gave me a hug and made me feel loved. She told me it's normal to get sad sometimes. I gave her a genuine smile and knew I didn't have to hide my pain from her. She held my hand and we went back out to finish watching the game together. At the time, I didn't have an answer to why I was so sad but having a friend to be there to talk to helped immensely and made me feel less alone, but now I better understand that I was experiencing major depression and have developed a skill-set to help me whenever I am feeling this way. I have learned to lean on my friends and family, to see a psychiatrist and listen to their advice, to take my medication, and to implement coping skills that help to distract me from my emotional pain.

Dear God

I had a relationship with God from a very young age. A special memory I have as a child was praying with my dad before bed. He'd come into my room at night and say a short prayer. He would then go on and ask me, "Who else should we pray for?" He stayed by my side as we listed off every family member, teacher, and person I knew. We even prayed for all the animals. He was patient with me and taught me that prayer doesn't need to be like it is at church; it didn't have to just be scripture and rituals. I could talk to God like I was talking to a friend. That's how my relationship with God began and grew.

My parents took me and my sister to a Catholic church most Sundays when I was young. Some days we would goof off in the pew while my mom and dad hushed us to be quiet, but as I got older, I did my best to listen to what the priest had to say. One thing about young children is that they have big imaginations. That is why so many of them believe in Santa Clause and the Tooth Fairy; at that age everything and anything feels possible. I was very literal as a child and an overthinker. I listened in church about how if you abide by certain Catholic rules and choose Jesus as your savior, then you would eventually end up in heaven with all your loved ones forever. I wanted to go to heaven one day. I wanted to be good enough so God would take me.

When I was about seven or eight years old, I would say my prayers every night and lay in bed and wonder about the concept of forever. Forever is a long time, and, if you think about it, it's almost hard to wrap your head around; even more so as a little kid. I remember lying there and having panic attacks thinking about it. I would need to stand up and walk around because I would get lightheaded. *What am I going to do forever in a never-ending place? How can forever have no end? What if I don't like it there? I will never be able to leave.* These were serious concerns for that age too.

I voiced these questions and stresses to my parents and they did what they could to console me. I would wake them up late at night crying because I just could not fathom the concept. I needed to understand. They were at a loss of what to do. I would lie next to my dad and we would listen to old murder mysteries on his radio. It distracted me from my fears and it felt comforting to sleep with my parents when I was little. The panic attacks and fear of "forever" lasted about a year. During this time, my parents reached out to a couple of people at church and even my third-grade teacher to ask for advice. It was a big deal in our family for a while. I could tell it caused my parents pain to see me experience so much panic and anxiety. I've often wondered if these panic attacks were early signs of mental illness or if it triggered mental illness later in life.

Kylie and I attended Monday night religion classes together at our Catholic church from a young age until our confirmation in high school. In classes, we read scripture and would talk through the meaning of it with our teacher. In all honesty, you could find Kylie and me laughing half the time at an inside joke. We got in trouble and were even separated a few times. I did my best to be a good Catholic and do what I could to live like Jesus Christ. I wanted to be as good of a person as he was.

This is why, as I lay in bed in the winter of 2012, I could not understand why I was not happy. I had done all the things I thought a good Catholic girl could do at my age. I really tried to be a good enough person. As I prayed harder and harder for God to make the pain go away, I felt worse because he wasn't fixing it. I started to question if he even wanted me. *What if my pain was a punishment because I was a bad person?*

Dancing Away the Darkness

My parents are some of the most supportive people. One thing I love about them is they always let me choose my own path, even if that means making a mistake. When I was little they put me in about every sport and some music lessons because they wanted me to pick my own passions. They never told me what to be or what to wear.

Of course they were my parents, so there was discipline. They rarely used it though because I was such a well-behaved kid. They encouraged me to lead my own life and be the special person I was meant to be. I have a good relationship with my mom and dad. I was always thankful they took the time to make it to most of my meets or games growing up. One of the reasons I was so reluctant about telling my parents about my depression and pain was because I didn't want them to be disappointed in me. Depression does that to you. It makes you feel like you're not good enough, like you're inadequate.

Rather than accepting the feeling that I was not good enough, I questioned whether there was something deeper that could explain how terrible I was feeling. I was in a sociology class the second trimester of my senior year. In class one day, the teacher spoke about how some people realize they are gay and attracted to the same sex. I didn't pay much attention until he began to share that young teens who are still in the closet can get very depressed and feel isolated and alone. *Could this be my problem?*

I was attracted to boys, I had no history of ever thinking otherwise. I liked kissing the one or two boys I had kissed in high school. But still, if being secretly gay is the reason why some young adults got depressed, what if this is why I was sad? *What if the reason I'm feeling depressed is because I'm gay or bisexual?* I knew something was wrong and I was grasping for an answer.

It was late December of my senior year in high school. As my depressive symptoms persisted, I began to struggle with short-term memory loss. It was more difficult for me to remember what I had just done, said, or what I needed to do next. I couldn't remember directions to familiar places–places we had gone all the time. After a basketball game we often ended the night at our favorite local restaurant. One night after a home game, I was driving Kylie and she pointed out that I took a wrong turn. I had to ask her which way the restaurant was. She looked at me like I was crazy for asking, as I was the one who mostly drove us. I felt dumb and embarrassed. She sensed that and laughed it off and told me the right way to go.

I later found out this was because of my lack of sleep. I was unable to focus at my best because my brain was so exhausted. My grades took a hit from this. Some days I would get a test and look down at the paper and just go blank. Around this time I was also feeling numb to emotions. I agreed to go on some dates with boys I was uninterested in just to try to feel something. We would have dinner or watch a movie, make out, and I just wouldn't text them back.

My relationships with my friends also suffered. I felt like a robot going through motions. When I hung out with friends it was hard to show any emotion because there were no emotions there. I felt like I was just existing. I was often known as the clumsy, goofy friend prior to dealing with depression. I could easily laugh at myself when I made a mistake and almost always had a smile on my face while around my friends because they brought so much joy. During this time, I wanted to still appear fun and goofy around my friends but I couldn't gauge humor anymore. I felt so hollow. Nothing was funny to me. Fake laughs and smiles can only get you so far. They weren't genuine, and I believe my friends could sense that. I could tell this hurt them, Kylie especially. She put a lot of effort into trying to keep me engaged.

I went on runs outside once in a while on the weekends. One day I was running down one of the trails in my hometown. There was a dust of snow on the ground and the sun was out. I ran hard and fast, feeling the cold air flow into my lungs. Running was one of the only things that could relieve the constant weight on my shoulders. That and hot showers and baths. As I ran I prayed to God and pleaded with him. I told God that if the issue were that I was truly gay, please let me realize and accept that so the bad feelings would go away. I was clawing for anything at this point. I would take long baths, submerging my entire body under the water and holding my breath. Relief would come when I wasn't breathing.

I began to carry a journal at school. During classes I would write inspirational quotes and positive comments about myself. I did it in an attempt to pull myself from the darkness. *You are strong. You are brave. You are fast. You are worthy. You are so very loved,* I would write.

As a senior, I was nominated for Snow Days queen. The entire bleachers were filled with all the kids in our school and almost everyone was wearing our school colors. One of the teachers stood in the middle of the floor trying to see what grade could cheer the loudest. There was so much exciting energy in the air.

I wore a beautiful blue dress and silver heels to the pep rally that day. Kylie and Kaitlyn helped me get ready in the bathroom before they called my name to walk out onto the gymnasium floor. They were so proud of me. I felt skinny and pretty. It was a good day. I felt happy so many people could have voted for me to be in that small, popular group. I walked out onto the floor with another boy in our grade and sat on stage. I wasn't picked as the winner, but I still felt special to be out there anyways.

I went to Snow Days dance that weekend with a group of girls, including Kylie and Kaitlyn. We were dressed in sparkly, sequined dresses and crimped one another's hair as we prepared for the evening. I still have pictures of us from that night. We went to the local diner for burgers and malts before the dance (I always ordered a chocolate-banana milk shake whenever we went), and then we headed out to the community center where the dance was held. Hip-hop and pop music played all night, and the dance was full of students from our school. There were times at the dance when I would go to the bathroom and look into the mirror and see sad eyes staring back at me. I smiled into the mirror and told myself this would be a fun night. We danced and laughed, and I got lost in the music on the dance floor. I felt numb but good. I was relieved to just move my body and let the music drown out my feelings.

A few nights after the dance I put that dress on again. It was in the middle of the night when everyone else in the house was fast asleep. I danced around my room attempting to dance away the darkness and feel the same numbness I had felt at the dance only a few nights prior. My attempt did not work, so I took the dress off and got back under my covers to try and get a decent amount of sleep before school the next day.

Exercising and moving my body was a therapeutic mechanism that helped relieve my unbearable pain during this time in my life. Having exercise as a part of my routine as an adult has been a great way to keep my body and mind healthy. However, moderation is key. In high school, I was over exercising as a way to suppress my feelings and in turn, was breaking down my body physically.

The First Time I Ever Thought about Suicide

The days began to get colder and darker in Minnesota with winter setting in. I was feeling more alone than ever and the weather did not help this.

In January, my dad began to notice some changes in me. Not only was it evident that I was at my lowest weight I had ever been, but he also began to notice my memory gaps.

He pulled me aside as I was walking out the door on my way to school one day in the morning and told me he sensed something was wrong. I stopped at the head of the stairs leading to our front door, curious, not knowing what I did. He said that when I would leave for school most days I would leave cupboard doors ajar, food on the counters, and sometimes even our front garage door wide open. He then pointed to all the ingredients and utensils I used to make my morning oatmeal that morning laying messily on the counter and one of the cupboard doors halfway open. He asked me how I could possibly be forgetting these things? He wasn't mad, just seemed concerned and a little bewildered.

I didn't know how to answer him. I had no idea these things were even happening. I rushed upstairs and cleaned up the counters, shut the cupboard doors, and put everything in its place. When he questioned me again, I made up something on the spot and shrugged my shoulders. I told him I was too much in a rush and that I would slow down and make sure everything was in its place before I left. I'm not sure if that answer was sufficient for him.

One thing no one tells you about depression: you don't just think up bad thoughts just because; they are intrusive. As nights passed, panic began to ensue because I could find no solution to rid me of my misery. Things were not getting better, they were getting much worse. The first intrusive thought hit me: I remember thinking to myself there was no hope for happiness again; that the only way to relieve my unbearable pain was to take my life. I sat straight up in bed and could not believe the thought had crossed my mind. *Had I really just thought that?* Anxiety and panic took hold. This could not be real. It felt like I was in a living nightmare.

I lay in bed each night squeezing our black toy poodle, Stanley. I was Stanley's person when I was in high school. In my hardest moments, Stanely would lay by my side and push himself up against me and let me hold him tight. If you knew Stanley, you would know he was a grumpy dog. He didn't like to be touched very often. But in my darkest times he let me pull on him and squeeze him, and he just lay there as I held him close to me. He made nighttime bearable. The intrusive thoughts were worse at night because I couldn't distract myself. I was forced to really feel my pain and loneliness. Terrible thoughts would come and I experienced thoughts of suicide almost every night since that first night. Even though I had suicidal ideation, I truly wanted to live. I would imagine myself going for a run and jumping off the bridge down the street, and then panic and try to push the thoughts away. They were so dark and scary. It truly was a waking nightmare. It was a living hell.

I needed to stay positive and continue to push these thoughts away. Kylie and I had begged our moms earlier in the year to take us on a spring break trip to celebrate our senior year together. It would just be us four. We booked a trip to the Dominican Republic that fall, and, in early March, we would be leaving for a week to soak up the sun and sip on virgin piña coladas on the beach. I could not let my bad feelings or thoughts get in the way of this trip. In January, I had lost interest in just about everything. I would go to the gym late at night and run long on the treadmill until the endorphins hit and I felt a sense of relief. I wanted to have the desire to go on this trip with Kylie and our moms, and I couldn't let Kylie down. She would talk about the trip almost everyday since the new year, and I wanted to have fun with her.

Basketball season began to wrap up. Often we would make it to the final game in sections against our main rivals. The winner of the game would advance to the state tournament. Every year for the last three years we came up short, but we had a chance this year. The bleachers were full of fans from both teams. During the game I ran up and down the court, shot the basketball into the hoop, and defended the ball and the opposing team. It took all I could muster to not walk off the court in the middle of the game because I was giving up on myself. I was tired of wearing a front I couldn't even recognize anymore. I remember the crowd sounding muted in my ears and not being able to keep track of what plays our team was running or even how to do them. I felt like I was moving in slow motion as I made my way up and down the court. At this point in time I was getting a maximum of five hours of sleep each night.

The game was close throughout the first three quarters, but we didn't win. Our team walked into the locker room defeated and sad. The girls were crying. I began to cry; not because we lost or because it was my last game I'd ever play, but because of the pain and distress I felt. I hugged my teammates and held on to each of them tight. To them, we were embracing the end of the season and another tough loss. To me, I was grasping onto any sense of relief. I couldn't care less that we lost. If anything, I was happy I didn't have to put any more effort into the sport. I realized at that point I needed serious help.

I opened up to my parents shortly after and told them I needed help.

"It's okay," they said. "We understand you've been stressed about college starting next fall and we know you have been really busy with school and basketball. It's okay! Take tomorrow off and stay home and relax."

"No," I said. "Something is seriously wrong with me. I am hurting and extremely sad. Everything feels difficult and I have no motivation."

They asked if I had thoughts of hurting myself. I lied and said, "No." I didn't want them to panic. One thing you have to understand about my parents is that they are very hard on themselves. If Ann or I are hurting, they tend to question if it is their fault as a parent. I couldn't let them down. It wasn't their fault. They were born in the 1960s in small towns. With no education in schools in the early 2000s about mental health issues, they had little to no knowledge about what I could possibly be going through.

Once everything finally came to light, they were hit hard with a truth they knew nothing about. It was not not anybody's fault. I was experiencing a severe mental illness that can only be treated if I had the correct professional care. They would come to blame themselves and that is not fair. Not fair at all. How would they know their daughter experienced suicidal ideation almost every day? From the outside, I looked like a happy kid. I hid my true feelings and emotions from them, from everyone, out of fear for what would happen to me. I didn't see any other solution.

I stayed home for a couple days and cried to my mom about not being good enough. I shared with her there was a possibility I was in fact gay. She laughed very hard at me. She said she knew for a fact I was straight. This didn't make me feel better even though I knew she was right. She was going to call the school and complain about my sociology class putting these thoughts in my head, but I talked her out of it.

She told me she would bring me to see a therapist if I wanted to. I agreed. Anything I could do to save my life at this point I was willing to try. We went to one or two sessions. I sat down and the therapist asked me why I was there. I told her something was very wrong with me and I thought I was messed up.

"What do you mean you're messed up?" she asked. I told her my big concern about being a lesbian. She asked if I had suicidal thoughts. I lied again. No one could know. She asked me a list of questions I can't quite remember and finally came to the conclusion I was not gay.

I left the clinic unsatisfied because she didn't solve my problem as to why I was depressed. She didn't give me a solution to relieve me from my constant pain. What I didn't understand was that sometimes people get depressed for no reason whatsoever. Mental illness does not discriminate by age, race, or ethnicity. It was not my fault like I strongly believed it was. Because it was determined that I was not gay, I accepted that my depression was caused because of me being bad and unworthy of God's love.

A close friend of my family passed away early that year. It was a shock to everyone. I had mowed his lawn throughout middle and high school. I remember sitting in the kitchen that day as my parents shared the news. I felt run down and gloomy. Even though the kitchen was bright, I felt like I had a gray veil over my head. It's like the lighting and coloring in the room was skewed to be more black, white, and grays. They turned to me and asked me how I felt and if I were okay. I sat there and felt nothing; no remorse or sadness. I felt numb to any emotion, as I had for weeks now. My parents noticed this and asked why I wasn't sad. I told them I was sick and didn't care. They were upset about this. My parents couldn't see how much I was struggling because from the outside I looked completely normal. I could tell they were frustrated with me and that hurt me. They told me I was being selfish. It felt like a punch to the stomach. They didn't mean to hurt me, but it was an awful thing to hear as a depressed person. I was just trying to get through each day and now I'm being selfish. *Why was I such a bad person?* I thought to myself.

Today, through education about bipolar disorder, my parents are so much more understanding when I'm experiencing episodes of depression. They never blame me or get upset. They listen to what I need and are patient with me.

We had our end-of-season basketball banquet a couple weeks after our final game. Each year at the banquet, the seniors give out gag gifts to the lower classmen. I remember this day like it was yesterday. I couldn't gauge humor, but I wanted to do my best at appearing funny when I announced the gifts for our younger girls and told stories from the season. Because I couldn't feel anything and couldn't scale emotions or humor anymore, one of the stories I told ended up being offensive and inappropriate. I didn't intend this at all. I was faking being goofy. The mother of the girl I was speaking of ended up confronting me at the end of the party. She was so angry and I honestly deserved what she said. I felt like such a bad person. *I am a terrible human being,* I thought. I told myself that everyone would be better off without me. I believed that I was a burden to others.

My Final Race

Now that basketball season was over, the time for spring sports had come. That meant track season. I was the fastest and fittest I had been in my entire life. I did not get to this point in a healthy way, as my disordered eating was still there. I was never diagnosed or treated for an eating disorder so I am unable to specify exactly what I was dealing with. What I do know is that it was definitely very unhealthy and at times, even when I wanted to stop, it was out of my control. I'm not sure if it was the fact I had been eating so little or because I was so mentally sick at this point, but my appetite ceased to exist. I struggled to eat. Many times throughout the day, I would forget to eat. I began to become light headed in gym class and at track practices.

We had our first indoor meet of the year at the University of Minnesota in the beginning of March. I completed the mile–eight laps–on an indoor track. I felt light and it was easy as I went around each curve with little to no effort. I crossed the line in first place with a time of five minutes and twenty seconds. It was faster than I had ever run a mile before. I couldn't even believe how fast I had run the race. My dad was there and I smiled because I could see how proud he was of me.

My coach told me I'd be his first athlete he'd ever had qualified to go to State in track. He believed in me and was proud I was his captain for the distance team. But I never made it to State that year. I didn't know it at the time, but I would never run a high school race again.

Just getting to school on time became an impossible task. I would crawl out of bed on my hands and knees in the morning and put on my clothes while sitting on the floor. I was in so much unbearable misery. I felt so much discomfort and distress.

By this point I was so sick that I was no longer running at the gym. My parents were seriously concerned with how skinny I was. My dad would plead with me to eat dinner. I sat at the table one night as he made me my favorite pasta. It was simple, just penne noodles with marinara sauce and alfredo sauce mixed together. It was a staple for Ann and me during most of high school.

I looked down at the bowl of food and felt sick. I forced a few noodles down, and my dad glanced at me with a concerned look on his face. My parents didn't know what to do. They are very private people so they did not open up to many others for help or advice.

I would walk out of classes during the day and call them crying and apologizing to them for being a failure and for letting them down. After I hung up I felt guilty for making them feel bad, so I would call back the next minute and apologize for saying those things and that I was okay and would get through this.

"You don't need to worry so much," I told them.

I could hear them whisper at night as they'd try and determine what to do. They were panicked and scared, rightfully so. My mom would lay with me at night and I'd ask her to hold my hand. My dad came into my room one night and asked what he could do for me. He told me he would do anything he possibly could to make me myself again and help me to be happy. I couldn't cry anymore.

I sat on his lap and took his face in my hands. I asked my dad if he would help me end my life because I was too scared to do it myself. It pains me to relive this memory and to write this on paper for others to see this. I broke my dad's heart that day, and I feel so awful about it. He wept and held me and made me promise him that I would never do that to myself.

He asked, "Don't you love us?" Of course I loved them. I loved them with all my heart. I didn't want to leave them, I didn't actually want to die. The depression and intrusive thoughts that came with it made me believe that that was the only way to make the pain stop. At this point my parents should have called 911, a mental health crisis hotline, or driven me to the emergency room. But they did not know that. They felt just as helpless as I was.

The Edge of my Breaking Point

My relationship with Kylie felt stressed and fake. I felt her sadness when she was around me. She attempted less to make me smile. Where had her friend gone? I was not myself. I didn't know who I was anymore. I felt like I was failing at life. My parents hadn't seen my grades yet, and I honestly didn't care. I was now averaging three hours of sleep a night.

It was the day before spring break. I had one final calculus test. Mr. Jensen set it in front of me that afternoon. I looked down at the equations and shapes on my paper and had no idea what I was looking at. I didn't bother to attempt to answer any questions or even make the answers up. I kept imagining myself walking out of class, to the front door of the school, out through the parking lot, and on to the street where I would get hit by a car. I would then push the thought aside because I could not let anyone be blamed for running me over. I couldn't ruin someone else's life. I waited for the bell to ring for the end of the school day. I handed my teacher a blank paper at the end of class, and he looked at me quizzically.

"Is everything okay?" he asked.

I told him a family member had just passed away and I had a lot on my mind and couldn't focus today. I promised him I would retake the test after spring break. He didn't seem convinced but didn't say anything and I walked out the door.

This is it, I thought. Deep down I told myself this was the last day I would ever spend in my high school. There was no way I would ever walk through the door again, not because I would take my own life, but because I would not be able to function any longer. It was physically impossible to carry on. I cleaned out my track locker at the end of the day, leaving nothing behind to inconvenience anyone from having to clean out my things later.

That night my parents came into my room and told me to make the best of the trip. All you have to do is lay in the sunshine, relax, and enjoy the beautiful weather. There is nothing to worry about. I actually believed them. Maybe the tropical climate would allow me to feel relief, and I could keep all this horror and darkness inside of me back in Minnesota.

I packed my suitcase that night. As I sat on the floor filling my bag, I needed to count out nine pairs of underwear for the trip. My short-term memory was so bad at this point that I would get to five and then would forget what number I was on. I had to restart multiple times. After what must have been five or maybe even ten minutes, I finally had the adequate amount of undergarments packed away in my suitcase to last me the nine days.

The next morning my dad picked up Kylie and her mom, Sue, to drive us to the airport. The car ride felt awkward. I was hopeful that what my parents said about going to a new place would make me feel relieved. We got to the airport, checked our bags, and began to head towards the security checkpoint. That's when it hit me. I can not run from this feeling. It is a part of me and wherever I go it will go. *I will always feel this way*, I told myself. I pulled my mom aside and asked her to take me home. She continued to insist that the sunshine and beach would be good for me. I nodded my head and tried really hard to believe her. I boarded the plane.

Up to this point, my parents had taken me to multiple therapy sessions and to a few doctors to try to understand why I was not feeling myself. Unfortunately, nobody was able to identify what the future held for me as I boarded the plane to the Dominican Republic. It was a very difficult and mentally draining time for my mom and dad.

From my parents' perspective, it would have been helpful to have someone complete, or even suggest, a mental health evaluation in order to dig deeper into my change in demeanor. As they have told me, they were never informed by any of the doctors or therapists that there was any reason to be alarmed. Though it seems we have come a long way with mental health awareness since this time, I don't think there is a clear cut way to navigate these situations as a parent. The answer may not always be as simple as doing X, Y, Z. However, creating a space for conversation and obtaining appropriate resources is key in the early stages and could help guide families down the road.

The Spring Break that Never Was

I only remember bits and pieces of the plane ride. I remember sitting next to Sue and crying and telling her that I had let my friends and family down. She seemed confused and looked very concerned. I think my mom had mentioned to her that I was struggling with anxiety or something along those lines. While I spoke to Sue, my mom sat with Kylie.

I remember the resort. It was beautiful and smelled of tropical flowers and salty ocean air. We got there early that same day. Kylie and I swam in the ocean, drank a virgin tropical, frozen drink, and lay by the pool. There was awkwardness between us, I had not been myself for months now. I pretended to sleep by the pool, feeling suffocated by the overwhelming physical and mental pain. We went up to the hotel room to get ready for dinner. Kylie and I showered together in our swimsuits to get the salt water off before we changed into our nighttime clothes. She washed my body and hair, taking care of me. It was so nice, and I don't know how she knew that I needed that.

We went to dinner, and I remember keeping busy by forcing myself to eat in order not to have to talk. I forced food down my throat. At this point, I think everyone could sense that something was very wrong. The lack of sleep over the last few weeks was causing me to get confused. I wasn't thinking straight and it was hard to string sentences together. That night we went back up to the hotel room and I was at my breaking point. My mom suggested I talk to Sue privately to try to explain how I was feeling. Kylie and my mom sat in the room as I talked with Sue in the hallway. I imagine that Kylie couldn't take it because she came into the hallway early in the conversation to find Sue and me sitting on the floor. I wasn't making sense. We discussed that it might be a good time for all of us to go into the room and talk everything out. They sat me down on one of the beds and asked what was wrong. In distress, I broke down and told Kylie and Sue all the terrible things I believed about myself. I told them that God didn't love me, that I was a bad person, that all my smiles and laughs were fake, that I was fake. I told them that I felt like I had a demon in me.

Sue began to cry and Kylie held my hand. I told them that I was going to die. At this point in my journey, I had no intention of committing suicide as I had promised my dad, but it obviously wasn't clear to my mom, Kylie, and Sue. They panicked as I lay on the bed. What I meant was that I was so starved, sleep-deprived, and felt so extremely terrible that I was just going to die from natural causes. There was no way I could carry on.

Something happened at this point, but I only remember fragments. I had my first psychotic episode. For those who do not know what that means, I lost touch with reality. I would later come to find out that at this point my mom got on the phone with the airlines and called my dad to find a way to get me home ASAP.

I became very paranoid. I truly believed that there was a demon living inside me and that my mom, Kylie, and Sue were out to get me. I believed they knew what I was thinking. Apparently at one point I was shoving bed sheets into my mouth to the point where Kylie had to hold down my arms. We went to bed that night, and I could tell everyone was wide awake. They were most likely fearful that I would hurt myself, but I believed they were fearful of me.

As I lay in the bed in my deranged reality, I began to hear thunder outside. I could hear people banging on the door and walls of our hotel room and feel the room shaking. Bad people were coming to get me and take me away. It felt so real at the time that there is no way you could have convinced me otherwise. I wanted to be good. I didn't want this demon to live inside of me. I needed to get rid of it and save my mom and dear friends that were with me.

A voice in my head told me I should jump out the balcony window. That this would rid me of the demon and save the ones I loved. I got out of bed and made my way to the sliding glass door. My mom got up and ushered me back towards the bed. I remember lying on the bed and screaming.

Men came into the room to try and calm me down. I didn't know these men. I was slashing and kicking and they could not control me. I didn't want them to hurt me. I don't know how much time passed before I remember feeling calm and them leaving the room and my mom telling them I would be okay. I think these people were there to help me so I wouldn't hurt myself but I don't quite remember. I fell asleep briefly.

The next morning I sat quiet against the bed frame with nothing to say. I felt exhausted, sleep deprived, and tense. I couldn't decide if I should fear my travel partners hurting me or try to save them.

Were they going to hurt me?

As I sat there and the others moved amongst the room in whispers I noticed something quite strange. Before we left, Mom and Sue had packed our suitcases with a handful of plastic water bottles. We were told not to drink the local water, so we brought our own water with us.

As I sat there, I was amazed to see the multiple water bottles were spread throughout the room, falling off the dressers onto the floor. One after the other they fell. It was clear as day. No one was touching them. I could even hear them hit the floor. How were my travel partners making this happen? Was it a trick?

Obviously this wasn't really happening but I truly believed the hallucinations that were being processed in my head. As I relive this through my writing, I still can't believe how scary and dark the mind can be. If you would have told me six months prior that these things would actually happen, I would have laughed at you and told you that you watch too many movies. But there I was. It was my reality.

After a while my mom asked me to get up and change my clothes. She told me we were going home. I listened to her and put on a pair of jean shorts and a t-shirt. Our suitcases were packed and

32

we headed down to the front lobby to get in the van that would take us to the airport. I felt relieved. They were going to help me feel better.

As we walked down the stairs to the grounds of our hotel, I thought about asking my mom and Sue who the people were that were pounding on the walls, and how the hell did they make the water bottles fall onto the floor without touching them? I guess I thought they'd share their trick with me at a later time. It was odd; there was no rain on the ground from the thunderstorm.

In the van on the way to the airport, I held Kylie's hand and my mom said she had something that would help me and she handed me a little white pill. I didn't know what it was. Instead of just asking, my psychotic self believed that the pill would rid the demon from my body. They were on my side! They were trying to help me. I took the pill happily. I remember boarding the airplane. I remember sitting in my seat next to my mom and Sue. And then I remember waking up.

Cherish

When I woke up, I was in a wheelchair being pushed off the plane. We went down a long hallway and came out to a big wall with writing in multiple languages that I didn't understand. My stomach sank. My mom and friends weren't trying to help me; they brought me to a foreign country to live out my days as a bad person. I could not believe I had been tricked! They wheeled me past customs and through the strange airport.

Now, what was actually happening at this time is that we landed in the Atlanta, GA airport and the writing on the big wall read "Welcome to the United States" in multiple languages because we had just flown in on an international flight. We were here to make a connecting flight home to Minneapolis where my dad and Kylie's dad would be waiting for us. What my mom had given me was Valium, a sedative that helps treat anxiety. While we were in the Dominican Republic, my mom called home to try and get me a prescription medication. She was unable to since we were out of the country, but a family doctor told her what to get me. Sue raced down to a pharmacy down the street from the hotel and purchased the Valium while Kylie and my mom stayed with me in the hotel room. It was in a small, clear bag and was not labeled. It actually didn't even require a prescription like in the United States. It was a shady, run-down pharmacy in our resort with limited hours. My mom and Sue didn't have many options though and were in need of something to calm me down. My mom, Sue, and Kylie had been doing everything in their power to get me home safely, so I could be admitted for adequate treatment. Of course, I didn't understand this. We never made the connecting flight from Atlanta to Minneapolis.

After we went through customs, we were making our way through the "foreign" airport. I decided that I would go off on my own and deal with this demon in my own way. I leapt out of the wheelchair and began to run through the airport, away from my mom and Sue. It must have been fate because as I was running past the bathrooms, Kylie stepped out and grabbed me. She tackled me to the ground. *How did she know to be there?*

I remember laughing at the fact that I couldn't get away from them. I don't recall this, but Kylie said I was laughing hysterically. She looked me in the face and took hold of my cross necklace that was around my neck and held it up to my face; she said something around the lines of "remember who you are."

Mom and Sue had caught up to us and sat me down on a chair as passersby called for help. I sat there and said nothing. I removed my cross necklace, placed it in Kylie's palm and told her to keep it safe for me, expressing in short that I could no longer wear it. Apparently my mom had also called for help as well.

Eventually paramedics came and attempted to strap me down in order to safely get me into the ambulance. I don't remember what happened next. Trauma does that to you, blocks out bad memories. Kylie later told me that I fought off at least three grown men as they worked to restrain me. She told me I even bent needles and ripped through straps that they were trying to use to calm me down. I can't imagine being as strong as she says I was, under 115 lbs, malnourished, sleep deprived, and out of my mind. I guess adrenaline can make you do crazy things when you're fighting for your life.

I woke up in a hospital bed surrounded by nurses and doctors. My sweatshirt had blood stains from the needles I fought off. A nurse came in and asked me to take all of my jewelry off. I did as she requested. She asked me why I was there and what happened. It was hard to remember and I felt confused. I told her that I had been on vacation, that there was a demon living inside me, and that my mom was trying to kill me. She nodded as she scribbled notes and told me that they were going to take care of me.

My mom came into the room. She was the last person I wanted to see at the time. I still believed she was plotting to hurt me and didn't want me anymore. She came over and kissed me on the head and asked if I would please sign some documents so that she could help with my treatment. This sounded like an awful idea. Legally I was an adult and she would not be able to have any knowledge of my hospitalization stay if I did not give her consent. It took a lot of pursuing, but I agreed, reluctantly, to allow my mom to be able to help me.

The rest of what I am going to share with you is my reality. I'm not sure if it actually happened, but they are fragments of memory in my mind. The nurses moved me into a new room. It was scary. No one looked like me. Some people had crazy hair, some were talking to themselves. I was handed a bed sheet that smelled strongly of bleach. I sat down in an uncomfortable chair with very little padding. The walls and floors of the room I was in were painted white and the ceiling lights were so bright. At this point I was coming in and out of reality. I was horrified by what had happened within the last twenty four hours. What had I done? What had I said?

I was so ashamed.

I curled up into a ball on my chair and forced myself to sleep. I told myself that I was in a nightmare and if I fell asleep I would wake up in my bed in Minnesota. I would wake up, feel horrified that I was still here, and sleep again. I finally got to a point where I could no longer force sleep upon myself. I became irritated. I wanted to leave and go home.

I walked to the main door and asked the men guarding the door if I could please see my mom. They said, "No." I was getting more frustrated. They couldn't just keep me in this room forever. I attempted to push my way past them, and they picked me up on either side and strapped me face down by my hands and feet onto a bed that also smelled of bleach.

I kicked and screamed and yelled for I'm not sure how long. Finally a nurse approached me, pulled down my pants, and stuck a needle in my butt cheek. I remember feeling a sense of calm wash over me, and I fell asleep.

I woke up in a room with two hospital beds in it and a closet without a door. I could see that there were cameras on the ceiling.

There was a stack of papers sitting on the night stand beside me. The first page had a large picture of a cross on it and had a question on it with something along the lines of 'Why are you here?' I picked up a pen and wrote in large letters, 'myself.' I stood on the bed and held the paper up to the camera. A nurse came into my room and told me it was time to eat.

I followed her into a hallway that led to a medium sized room with a large table. I was the only one there. There were posters on the walls with inspirational quotes and people smiling. I remember eating grits and chocolate chip cookies. I don't remember what else.

The next day they told me that someone was here to see me. I made my way through the strange, eerie hallways. I was still wearing my bloody clothes as well as a hospital gown in the front of me and a hospital gown in the back in order to cover myself. I later found out that they had isolated me and attempted to cover me so I would not be preyed on by the other male patients. This had been an issue there before and later I found out a girl was raped onsite by another patient. Looking back I realize how unsafe of a place I was in, even though I did need psychiatric care. I had not showered in over three days. I passed more scary people, strange people, sad looking people. We ended up in a small room.

There sat my mom and my uncle, John. The one who lives in Minneapolis, MN. *How did he get here?*

I looked at my mom suspiciously, still not knowing if I trusted her. John told me he was here to help me and my mom. He said I had three simple tasks that would get me back home. "Eat, sleep, and listen to the nurses." I didn't say anything but nodded.

My mom bought me a small pack of Reese's Peanut Butter Cups and a stack of brand new clothes so I didn't have to wear the hospital gowns anymore. She even gave me her shoes. They weren't very useful because she had to take the shoelaces out of them for safety purposes. I put them on briefly, but ended up wearing socks for the rest of my stay at Cherish.

A man took me and my mom to a separate room and told me I was in a psychiatric facility and asked me how I would like treatment.

The options were religious treatment or standard treatment. I was shocked. Were they going to try and do an exorcism on me? Was this God's way of taunting me? At this point in my journey I did not want anything to do with God because I thought he did not want anything to do with me.

I quickly picked the standard treatment plan. My mom introduced me to a nurse. Her name was Jen. She smiled at me and told me she was there to help and answer any questions. She said she worked the day shift.

My mom and John visited me everyday, even when I didn't want them to. I never actually comprehended that I was there to get treatment so I could safely go home. I figured it was a place for insane people where we were sent to live out our days.

After they left, I changed into a pair of clean clothes without showering. There was nowhere to shower that I was aware of. I went into a room that looked like a living room. I sat amongst strange people. A woman came in and told us that we were going to watch a movie and that she was there to guide us to be better people. I didn't trust anyone. For all I knew, they were involved in banging on the walls back in the hotel room in the Dominican Republic.

After we watched a movie it was time to take our medicine. There was a little window where we all lined up. When it was my turn I told the woman my name, and she handed me a cup full of different colored pills. I didn't know what they were trying to give me. I spit the meds in the garbage and the nurse yelled at me. I didn't spit them out because I wanted to be bad or because I didn't want to take it. It's hard to explain, but in my psychosis I thought I deserved to be punished. By making them upset and not doing what they said, it was like I would get what I truly deserved. I believed that I was bad and unlovable.

This was one of the lowest moments in my life. They told my mom and John what I had done and he reminded me, "Eat, sleep, and listen to the nurses."

After that day I did as they said. I took the meds as they said and ate when they said. The medication made me extremely tired and constantly hungry. No matter how much I ate, I could never feel full.

Each night, the nurses and help staff would come into my room every hour with a flashlight to check on me. It was scary because I didn't know why they were doing that. Every morning someone would come in and say that they needed to take a blood test. For at least three days straight they took a new blood sample.

I walked up to Jen one day to ask her a question. She told me she could help me "in a little bit." I was so exhausted and heavily medicated that I could not keep my eyes open and the staff had locked each of the patients' doors so we would not lay down and sleep in any of the beds. I laid on the ground and fell asleep waiting for her to come and speak with me.

They eventually moved me into a new area that had a nicer room and its own shower. I could not wait to shower. The bathroom was very simple with very few nobs and no toilet seat (nothing to harm you or anyone with). I stripped off my clothes and looked at my body in the mirror with horror. I was covered in bruises and needle marks. It had felt like a dream that I had been poked in the bottom with a needle. But as I turned around and stared at my backside, there it was. A small bruise where a needle had been. The other bruises throughout my body were from me fighting off all of the men who were trying to help me back in the Dominican and while at the Atlanta airport.

The shower felt amazing. I stood there for at least ten minutes letting the water run through my hair and down my body. Even my bathroom had a camera in it. I didn't care if they saw me naked. I showered, changed, and flipped the camera off on my way out the door.

I stayed in this hospital for two weeks. Everyday I would walk up to the front desk, and they would ask for my name. I couldn't have anything in my room. Not even a toothbrush or a hair brush. I also had to return everything after I used it. The only thing I was allowed to have in my room were my clothes and the Reese's Cups my mom would bring me. It made me really irritated that everytime I requested something they asked for my name again, no matter how many times I went up there. They obviously knew my name was Kate. Because they didn't seem to sense my annoyance, I decided to play a game with them. I began to tell them a different name every time they asked. The first time I did it I walked up to ask for a snack. I smugly said my name was Liz. I even ripped off the hospital band around my wrist that said my name as if I were actually going to trick them. They didn't say anything, scribbled some notes, and handed me a pack of crackers. I was unsatisfied that it didn't seem to annoy them.

I spoke to Kylie on the phone once in a while. There was a lot of awkward silence and I had no idea how to address my best friend after all the events that had happened. She said such positive things to me and about me and made me promise her I would do what I could to get back home to Minnesota so we could graduate together later in the spring.

Everyday my mom and John would visit. My mom would always sneak in Reese's Peanut Butter Cups because she knew they were my favorite. John looked me in the eye one day and told me that he promised that one day he'd be dancing with me at my wedding. I scoffed because I did not believe him. I was never having a wedding. I was never leaving this place alive. He didn't laugh and said he was going to keep his promise.

I began to keep a journal where I would write my feelings and draw during the day.

April 2nd, 2013 journal entry:

> *My entire life I've strived to be the best I can be. Whether it's through running, water skiing, basketball, homework, cleaning my room, etc... I was/am always going to give my best effort through hard work and determination. I always knew I was different from my friend, especially when it came to emotions. Being accepted has always been enough. I want to go home so badly, but I feel stuck and don't know how to help*

> *myself. I miss Ann, Dad, and Stanley, and I don't know if I'll ever have a chance to see them again. Having my mom here gives me comfort. I know she said I need to help myself... and I'm trying but I don't think I deserve anyone's help.*

I smoked my first and only cigarette in the mental hospital. I was still not myself and had a very pessimistic mindset. I didn't care what happened to me as I believed this hospital was now my forever home.

On breaks between group therapy or eating they would allow us to walk outside in this crappy little gated area with little to no grass. All the women took smoke breaks. I would often go outside with them and let my body feel the sunshine. I missed my family cabin in northern Minnesota back home. Instead of seeing a beautiful sunset I was surrounded by gray walls, a tall fence, and a cracked, cement, patio floor with weeds poking through. I thought to myself that this little cement slab was the closest I'd ever get to sunlight again, so I had to make the best of it.

One day I asked one of the ladies for a cigarette. I sat outside with them on a cracked, plastic chair and smoked half a cigarette. It tasted gross but I didn't care.

I spent Easter in Cherish Hospital. They had an Easter Egg hunt for the tenants with candy-filled eggs. It was not the same as spending Easter at the cabin with my grandparents and family and that made me sad.

If you told me then I would have the life I have now, I honestly would have never believed you.

Eventually, I hit a breakthrough. I wanted to go home. I needed to go home. No more games. I asked the nurse to summon my mom and John. My mom came in not too long after that, and I told her I was so extremely sorry for what I put her through. I told her I loved her so much. She told me that my dad was on his way, and he was going to take us home. I almost didn't believe her. Was it possible I wouldn't die in this sad place? I felt optimistic and waited patiently for my dad to arrive.

The next day, there he was. He walked in with open arms and held me close. I could tell he was trying not to cry. I'm sure he was in shock about everything that had happened to me over the last few days. I felt so much love seeing him, but I was also embarrassed. I felt extreme shame for what I had done and said and believed. I told him I was so sorry.

I showed my dad the pictures I had drawn in my free time, and he brought me pictures of me and my friends and family from home. He showed me a picture from the previous Thanksgiving–I was smiling next to my grandpa and he had his arm around me. He showed me a picture of Ann and I at the state meet grinning at the camera together. One of the pictures was of Kylie, Kaitlyn, and I at one of our high school's football games wearing our school colors with warrior paint smeared across our cheeks, and he also had a picture of me water skiing at my grandparents cabin. We played a few hands of cards.

He asked, "Did you actually smoke a cigarette? Why would you do that?"

I smiled and felt embarrassed. I said I did it because everyone else was. "Look where I am. Why the hell not?"

He laughed nervously and I laughed about how absurd it was that perfect me would ever do such a thing. They told me we would head home tomorrow as soon as my discharge papers were ready. I was diagnosed with major depressive illness.

Home

We left the hospital the next day to head to the airport. I could not believe it as I stepped onto the plane after the flight attendant called, "boarding for Minneapolis, Minnesota." This was real. This was happening. I was going to be able to have a normal life at home again.

Throughout the plane ride I sat in between my parents, smiling and asking them if it were really true. I would list off my home address and ask them if that was where we were headed. They would smile, squeeze my hand, and answer yes.

We landed in Minneapolis later that spring day. The weather was sunny and bright, all the snow had melted. My dad drove us home, and I walked into the house to find my sister and Stanley greeting me. I was so excited and I hugged them both. Stanley was jumping up and down and giving me kisses. I almost started crying as I gave my sister a hug. She walked me into my room and told me the family had gotten me a welcome home gift. There was a new pair of running shorts sitting on my bed. I was so happy.

While I was away, my parents had been in contact with the school and had lined up a local therapist and psychiatrist for me to see. I would begin going to school again, only for half days, and I was not going to be competing on the track team. I met with my psychiatrist for the first time. He was a nice, older man named Dr. Anderson. He mainly saw adolescents but agreed to take me in since I had turned eighteen not too long ago. I was prescribed Risperidone, Cogentine, and Zoloft for medication. I didn't know anything about them, and I did not do research or ask questions. I simply/just did as he said.

Many Americans take Zoloft, one of the most common antidepressants. Risperidone, on the other hand, is an older drug which is used to treat schizophrenia and psychosis. That is what I was taking back in Georgia. The side effects were terrible. After I had returned home, I experienced a long list of symptoms. I needed to get reading glasses because it caused blurriness. It was extremely hard to wake up in the mornings and get my brain working. I was always hungry and thirsty. The medication causes dry mouth, so when I was out on my runs I couldn't produce saliva. After a while I began to lactate–another symptom. I took the Cogentine in order to make the side effects of the Risperidone more mild. Cogentine decreases the effects of muscle stiffness and sweating.

April 10th journal entry:

> *The voices in my head are calm and I don't want to hurt myself. I still get very confused at times. Physically I feel sore, somewhat weak, and I have blurred vision when I try to read things up close when I don't have my glasses on. I am trying really hard to get back in the swing of things. Overall I feel much better than when we left for the Dominican Republic.*

I got together with my uncle John frequently. We would go on walks and, even though I didn't open up much about my feelings, he was kind and listened intently and wanted to help. Having him with me in my lowest times brought us closer than we had been before.

I headed back to school for the first time in a month. I was scared of all the questions I would get and nervous to go back to my old life acting like nothing had happened. My parents told me to go to the school counselor if I needed anything at all; I could sit in her office any time.

Kylie was by my side. I could not believe she still wanted to be my friend after all she had seen. But there she was. I was embarrassed about everything that had transpired on our trip, but she didn't blink an eye or pass any judgment. She gave me a hug and a smile and helped me manage my new schedule at school. She told me to text her at any time during the day if I needed anything.

Because I already had all my credits to graduate, I didn't need to go back full time, and I didn't need to take my advanced classes anymore. I spent the first hour of my day in study hall and my last few hours in classes like art and cooking. By 11:30 everyday, I would head home.

Strangely enough, I didn't get many questions from my classmates about where I had been all this time, or the most awkward question: "How was your trip?" Thankfully no one asked for details about our spring break trip. Kylie protected me from all of the awkward questions and stares. I later came to find out that she had told everyone our trip was good and fun. She kept it short and sweet. She even showed my classmates some pictures that we took the first day. I am so thankful she helped me with my transition back. The teachers asked very few questions and were there if I needed help with anything.

It felt so good to be home. Still there was a lot of awkwardness in our household. I didn't know how I would gain back the trust of my parents. I didn't want them to see me as scary or a ticking time bomb. My parents went above and beyond for me; they wanted me to live a normal life. They took me to Mayo Clinic in Rochester to get a second opinion. The doctors told us they don't have a straightforward answer to why this happened. I would need to live my life and experience more things before I could get an accurate diagnosis.

I began going to see a new therapist, Jennifer. She was a nice lady and my first experience in therapy. For an hour twice a week I would sit in her office, awkwardly, not really knowing what to say. You would think I would have a lot to talk about, but I did not feel comfortable opening up. She had my hospitalization records from Cherish so she knew about the events leading up to my admittance to Cherish. I would sit there each session and she would continue to tell me it would be okay and that all of this was not my fault. She was trying to console me. It took me five years to find a therapist I ended up trusting and building a relationship with. The reason it took me so long was because I didn't put the effort in when I did meet with future therapists. I never let myself reflect very much on my past and let myself be vulnerable. I wish I would have attempted to open up and had pushed my embarrassment aside. One thing that is so great about therapists is that they are there to create a non-judgemental environment and what you share with them is confidential.

While all of this was going on, my sister was in the dark. She did not know what happened over spring break or in Georgia. She was not aware of all that happened leading into my psychotic episode. I'm sure she sensed something initially, but she was only fourteen, a teenager herself. Looking back I understand why my parents didn't tell her much and wanted to protect her from the truth. *What would they say? Kate is in the hospital because she lost her mind?* I think they did tell her I was sick and that was about it. The main reason why my dad did not come to Georgia when I was there was so he could stay with Ann as she was, of course, in school. When he flew down to get me, she stayed at a friend's house. I didn't end up sharing my story with Ann until I was in college. She let me know it was confusing for her and frustrating. She knew something was wrong but didn't like that she wasn't told about it. I honestly think she struggled a bit from feeling left out and that hurts me. She was thankful I told her the truth, and today I am very open with her about how I am doing.

Just because I was out of the hospital, taking medication, and seeing a therapist, it did not mean I was healed. I was still very depressed and extremely ashamed and embarrassed. After going through what I had gone through, my brain was injured. I had a lot of recovery to do. I was functioning and back in my old life, but I wasn't necessarily happier. I felt like I was still just existing and going through the motions.

However, it was a relief that I had people that had known what I had gone through who spoke very optimistic of my recovery back to a normal, happy life. nother symptom of both Risperidone and Zoloft is suicidal thoughts. It is very common to have suicidal ideation after your first hospitalization stay.

My Suicide Attempt

I remember very little of this day, I'm not sure why. I had only been in school for a week or two since I had gone back.

I was sitting in the study hall for the first hour, writing. I remember writing two letters, one addressed to Kylie and one addressed to my parents. I remember them being long, but no matter how hard I try I have no idea what either of them said.

I believed that by doing this I was saving my family embarrassment and pain from having me be around them. As their daughter, I believed that I was insane and a disappointment. I wanted to give Kylie her letter before I left that day. I texted her to meet me at my locker before second period. I quickly texted back 'nvm' because I didn't want her to tell my parents what I was about to do.

I'm not sure why I did this, maybe because I didn't think he'd be there, but I called my dad and told him I was going home early for the day because I was having a bad day. He said okay and told me to drive home safely. I don't recall my drive home or what I was thinking. I pulled into the second garage and shut the garage door. I sat there for a moment, remembering the baths I would take and the sense of relief I felt when I wasn't breathing. I wasn't frightened. I was calm.

I folded up my letters so they sat propped up on the steering wheel of my vehicle and I laid back and shut my eyes as the car engine ran, letting the carbon dioxide fill up the garage, the car, and my lungs. I don't know how much time passed until my dad walked into the garage. I quickly turned off the car and tucked my letters in my pocket. He didn't say much, but I followed him inside. Both my mom and dad were working from home that day.

Within minutes of me sitting down to eat lunch, my parents announced that they were going to be admitting me to a hospital in Minneapolis. I sighed sadly because I knew I had let my parents down again. I broke my promise to my dad—the most important promise. I agreed and got in the car, and they drove me to Johnson Emergency Room. I was silent the entire ride there. In the ER, they asked why I was there. I said nothing. My parents shared that they had witnessed me being suicidal. I excused myself to the bathroom and flushed my notes down the toilet. I was admitted to the psychiatric unit that day.

Johnson

Johnson was a huge step up from Cherish. It was clean and pleasant. I sat down with the main doctor there, and he told me that if I wanted to get better, I needed to tell him and the nurses all that I was feeling. I needed to be honest with them even if it was hard. This was a turning point in my treatment. I wanted to help myself. A person needs to accept that they want to get better and take action to do so. This stands true to this day. I had to take this step for myself; neither my parents nor Kylie could do it for me. No more games or smoke breaks or tricks. I was going to choose me. I deserved that. My parents and sister deserved that. Kylie and Kaitlyn deserved that.

I met with my doctor regularly to adjust my meds. I told them when I couldn't sleep, when I was having bad thoughts, what I was scared of. I told them my biggest fear was myself, my mind. I attended group therapy every day.

I eventually got access to the pass that allows you to leave the psychiatric health section of the hospital. At Johnson you would receive different level passes based on the progress you were making. This meant when visiting hours came I could walk throughout the hospital freely with my parents. My parents called and visited everyday, and I had the ability to call them at any time. It meant so much that they came to see me; I know they were on my side. They brought me pictures of happy memories, pictures of me with my family and friends doing the things I used to love. We hung them on the wall of my room I was staying in. They brought Kylie with them once. We all walked down to the main floor of the hospital and ate at the hospital's McDonald's. I ate ice cream and didn't worry about how many calories I was consuming.

Everytime I re-entered the psychiatric area, I had to take off my clothes, and they had to search me to make sure I wasn't bringing in any dangerous objects.

Kylie and I wrote notes to each other almost everyday, and my mom would be our delivery system. Those notes did so much for me, I still have some of them.

There would be times during the day where we would be able to bake, do crafts, color, or read. I often found therapy in drawing or coloring.

They allowed us to select our meals each day. Granted it was hospital food, but it was much better than the grits and canned green beans I was eating in Cherish.

I felt safe at Johnson and I actually enjoyed it there. I met some interesting people as well. Some were scary and strange, but there were a few who were kind. As I was sitting at the table one day reading a book, I saw a young woman with sad eyes being dropped off at the door by her husband, baby, and small child. Her husband kissed her and her son wrapped his arms around his mother's legs, and she held him tight. This woman ended up being my roommate. She told me that she had been dealing with depression all of her life, she must have been in her thirties. She had learned to live with it. She told me that the reason why she chose to admit herself to Johnson was because she was experiencing postpartum depression and she wanted to be the best mother for her children. She said that things do get better, and I believed her. She gave me hope. I remember thinking that if I ever had to be admitted while I was a mother, I would have that mindset and a supportive husband standing beside me.

I no longer look at psychiatric hospitals as bad places. The one in Georgia was not pleasant and I would never recommend anyone stepping foot in there. But there are really good ones out there. There is such a heavy stigma about having to spend time in one of these places, but Johnson saved my life. It was safe and allowed me to receive around-the-clock care.

When I was discharged after about two weeks, I was ready to go home. I understood that I would have to continue to keep working hard and listen to the professionals to help me get where I wanted to go, but living a happy life was a possibility. It wasn't easy. Frankly, it was hard as hell. When you leave the hospital, your life and how you live it becomes a choice again. I chose life.

Graduation

Going back to school after everything that had happened over the last couple months was extremely uncomfortable. I liked that no one asked me about where I was, but at the same time, I felt like such an outsider and out of place. I went through a very traumatic experience, not only over spring break, but also most of my senior year. Now I was put back into the environment and everyone (including myself) acted like nothing had happened and nothing had changed. I felt like the big elephant in the room. As I would walk through the school hallways, I could only remember the bad thoughts and the loneliness I had felt. I remember standing in the bleachers, looking down at the basketball court, and feeling so much resentment towards the sport and all the terrible pain and hopelessness I felt running up and down that court. I thought about all the fake smiles and laughter. I began to despise my highschool.

I went to prom that spring of my senior year. It is an event that everyone looks forward to attending in their high school careers. However, I had no interest in going. My parents and Kylie encouraged me to go, and soon after, I went shopping to find a prom dress with Kylie, Sue, and my mom. I picked out a dress in my favorite color purple. It was very beautiful but I felt a little awkward spending the day with Sue, Kylie, and my mom because the last time we were all together was on spring break. It was hard to not feel ashamed. They were all so kind and patient with me while I tried on my dress.

The day came, and I did my best to have fun. I felt awkward and it wasn't that enjoyable. I didn't have the same exciting and upbeat energy as everyone at the dance. I was so anxious and felt out of place. Kylie and Kaitlyn spent a great deal of time with me, encouraging me to dance with them. Looking back, I am happy that I decided to go. Even though I didn't feel like myself, I was in a much better mental state than before my diagnosis with major depression. I was in my healing process and I recall the feelings I felt were more so symptoms of my medication. My medication made me feel like I couldn't sit still at times and that caused me discomfort and anxiety. I must have been a bore to my date, as I didn't say too much, and I'm sure he could sense my demeanor. He was very respectful and kind and didn't prod me with questions about the last three months. He was also understanding when I said that I just wanted to go home after the dance had ended.

May 10th, 2013 journal entry

> *Today I only went to school for an hour. I felt very anxious... I needed to move around. I had to do something with my hands. I practiced putting them in my lap and that helped somewhat. I also felt like I had a pit in my stomach. I went home early, did some coping exercises and skills I learned from the therapist. Dad really helped me talk through my coping exercises. I went running and had tight and heavy legs. Could that be from my medication? By the end of the morning I felt relaxed and like myself again. Overall I hope that I am not a problem to Mom and Dad. I couldn't do this without their support.*

After a long and challenging three trimesters, I finished my senior year and got to celebrate graduation with Kylie, Kaitlyn, and my classmates. It did not feel like a celebration. I tried really hard to have fun but still felt anxious and crazy. I felt crazy because I had never heard of anyone else going through what I went through. I didn't even have a straightforward answer to what it was I did go through. I could feel the love of all the people around me that helped me tremendously but I wanted to be my old self again.

I told my parents that I did not want a party but they insisted upon it. They threw me a large, beautiful graduation party in our garage and backyard. My dad cooked up hamburgers and had one of those rollers where the hotdogs are made in bulk, like at a gas station. They were a huge hit. My grandpa and some other close family even drove to town to celebrate. They had no knowledge of what was going on in my life the last three months or where I had been, and my family kept it that way for a while. It felt good to see them. I don't remember much from the party because I was still being treated with Risperidone and it affects short term memory. That aside, I do remember it being a fun time. My favorite part was the end of the night when a group of friends from my high school sat around one of the tables and played games. We laughed and reminisced on the good memories. For the first time in months I forgot about the pain and the terror and sadness. I felt like Kate.

Freshman Year

As the spring and summer time went by, days began to flow and became less difficult. My relationship with my parents grew strong again. I was so grateful that Kylie still wanted to be a part of my life. I couldn't have gotten rid of her if I tried. We wouldn't talk about spring break of 2013 again for a few years.

Sue was just as supportive. I always felt a little ashamed around Sue after all that had happened. She was and had always been like a second mom to me growing up. She coached many of my sports and was always there to host sleepovers when I went to Kylie's. I wanted to make her proud.

My parents told me that I did not need to go to college and run cross country and track. They told me I could work somewhere in the Twin Cities and take a year off from school or take a few classes at the community college if I'd like. I appreciated that they didn't put pressure on me, but I was yearning to run. I wanted to experience college life, and, even if it were hard and scary, I knew I could do it.

I ran throughout the summer at my grandparent's cabin in northern Minnesota, my favorite place in the entire world. I bussed tables at the local restaurant down the street, ran, and spent time with my family. Things weren't the same as before, but they were definitely improving. The intrusive thoughts were gone.

In mid-August, I arrived at campus and my family was moving me into my dorm. It had only been four months since my stay at Johnson, but it felt much longer than that. I met my roommate, Kayla. She was a freshman too and a volleyball player for the school. She was very welcoming and we hit it off right away.

Only athletes and freshmen were on campus at this time. Classes didn't start for two more weeks but practices and freshman orientation were to begin the day after I arrived. My parents met my coach before leaving. With tears in my eyes, I gave my mom and dad a big hug and thanked them for all they had done to get me to this place. I was sad to see them go and somewhat frightened to navigate this independent life on my own without having them to lean on.

Classes were a challenge. My first class began at 8 a.m.; Intro to Statistics. I would try really hard in the morning to open my eyes even though I was so drowsy from the medication. I would tell myself if I went to the local coffee shop across the street and bought a latte, it would give me the strength to get to my first class and it would also be an enjoyable treat.

Getting to my first class for the first semester in college was a challenge everyday. I never felt fully awake until around noon. I would often take naps between classes and before practice would start. Kayla was always so nice and understanding when she would walk in and I'd be wrapped up in my blankets or when I would go to bed before 8:00 p.m.

My grades were nothing to write home about. I got my first D ever my first year of college. It was an intro to Microeconomics course/class. It was hard to focus, and I found the class to be uninteresting.

I ate more food than I ever had in my life to try and feel satiated. I never did. It was awful spending every waking moment hungry. If it weren't for running, I would have definitely gained a lot of weight.

My teammates were all very energetic and accepting and my coach, Cal, seemed good too. Runs were difficult. I was averaging fifty-five miles a week but the medication caused dehydration and stiff muscles and my legs always felt heavy. There was never really a run my freshman year that felt natural and easy like they had in high school. Some days it would take all I could muster to not stop in the middle of a run because my legs burned so badly with lactic acid. I told my doctor about my difficulty with my running and he told me that the Risperidone was the cause. He increased my Cogentine to help with the side effects of dehydration and stiff muscles.

I grew close with a few of the women on the team, and for the most part I was enjoying myself. One girl that I really hit it off with was Taylor. Taylor is one of the smartest and selfless people I've ever met. We ran together often and spent time together when we weren't in class or at practice. She was a talented runner and was going to school to pursue a degree in nursing, our college being known for their nursing program. A lot of graduates would end up getting jobs at well-known hospitals like Mayo Clinic after they graduated.

I was homesick most days. I would call my parents crying and tell them how hard school was and I didn't know if I could do it. They asked if I wanted to come home, and I would always say "No." I didn't want to give up. My mom would send me care packages with treats, Reese's Peanut Butter Cups, a note, and often money to buy my morning coffees.

Early in the fall, one of the older girls on the team, Jordan, asked me if I wanted to hang out with her and some of the other upperclassmen. They hosted bible study once a week and then ended the night with snacks and some games. It had been months since I had spoken to God. I didn't want anything to do with him. I was hesitant at first but decided to go.

Jordan met me at my dorm that evening, and we walked together down the lamp-lit street to the house that some of the girls were renting. She told me that she was really homesick her freshman year as well and promised it would get easier. She told me I could text her at any time and we could hang out together. It felt special hanging out with some of the older girls and having a person there who had felt the way I did. She made me feel included.

As weeks went by, I attended more bible studies. While I am a Christian and use the word "God" to describe a larger force in my life, I understand and respect that not everyone refers to that force as "God" or may not believe in a larger force at all. My experience was that when I opened my life back up to God, I became happier. Life became meaningful again.

I spoke with Kylie frequently. She was going to college in a different state. She wanted to be an occupational therapist. I would later find out that she decided to minor in psychology because she wanted to be educated so that she could help me and take care of me if need be.

I was chosen to race in Saint Paul at the Roy Griak Invitational, one of the largest and most famous Minnesota meets that year. Teams came from all over the country. We traveled to the University of Minnesota. On that day, many of my old teammates and coaches from high school drove to the course to watch me race. I was excited and proud to be there, but I dreaded the pain in my legs. Griak is a difficult race. The race is six kilometers and held on a golf course with many rolling hills. I waved to my parents and my high school coach at the start line.

Finally, the gun fired. The race had begun. I went out fast and ran alongside one of my teammates, Clara. Unsurprisingly, my legs felt like crap. I did my best to keep a good head on my shoulders and push through. It was a hard race, and I could feel the incline as I went up each hill. I eventually fell behind Clara. My brain began to fog. Only two hundred meters before the finish line, I collapsed. I tried to crawl but was too weak. A race official ran out and helped me walk off the course. I felt embarrassed that my high school coach and old teammates had witnessed me collapse and walk off the course before finishing. It was the only race in my seven years of racing that I did not finish.

The meet trainer took me into the medical tent and had me lay back and lift my legs up in the air against a chair. I was meant to keep them at a ninety degree angle to drain the lactic acid from my legs. It was extremely painful, almost unbearable. I continually lowered my legs in order to get relief, but she would come back and ask me to put them up again.

Coach Cal came and found me after the race. We went back to the team tent, and he gave me something to eat. He told me he wanted to speak with me, so we went on a walk. He told me he knew how talented I was, and he could see how much effort I was putting in. He knew I was on medication for something having to do with mental health but didn't know what it was. He stopped walking and looked at me. He told me that I needed to make a choice. The medication was obviously hindering my performance. I needed to choose if I wanted to stop running or if I could cut back on my meds. I was taken aback. It made me feel embarrassed because I truly was putting in so much effort. I told him that running was very important to me and I would see what I could do. Looking back, I realize that Cal did not know the extent of my condition, but I cannot wrap my head around the ultimatum that was presented to me. This is just another example of the lack of understanding around mental health and goes to show how certain words and reactions can impact if and how a person decides to get treatment.

I would head home at least once a month to see Dr. Anderson and adjust my medications. He was happy with my progress. It was actually his idea to decrease my medication a bit to see if I could relieve some of the side effects while still progressing.

I didn't drink or party much in college. First, I knew I wasn't supposed to drink on my medication and, second, our girls team was having a dry season. This meant we were not going to partake in drinking while we were training or competing. We would often go to the boys' cross country house on weekends and play games and listen to music while they drank. I didn't have time to date anyone and was uninterested. I was just trying to manage my new lifestyle and keep my grades up. Winter had come and I had a good group of friends.

Track season in college begins in late January. We would race indoors for about a month before the weather got nicer and then we moved outdoors. I continued to improve, decrease medication, and the side effects were lifting. Running became a little more bearable but still not like what it used to be.

January 29th, 2014 journal entry:

> *I had a very busy and productive day. I felt down. I*
> *know not everyday's gonna feel great, but it scares me*
> *when I feel down. I cried for no reason. It feels good to*
> *be back to school though. I absolutely hate and feel*
> *uncomfortable when I smell something that reminds*
> *me of the hospital in Atlanta.*

I shared with my coach that I was working to decrease my medication and I was seeing improvements. "I want to be here," I told him. "I choose running."

Once outdoor season was upon us, Cal let me know that he thought it would be a good fit for me to run in the steeplechase event. Steeplechase is a three thousand meter race with long racing hurdles and a water pit which you have to jump over throughout the 7.5 lap race. I would meet with him on the weekends, and we would practice clearing the water pit. For most of the hurdles I would jump over them without touching them, but for the hurdle with the water pit, I would need to put one foot on the hurdle and lunge myself over the water below. I ran a few races that season. It was challenging but I loved it. I was even chosen to race in the conference meet at the end of the year.

My parents came and watched that run. I felt strong as I cleared each hurdle. I remember it being difficult but I also remember feeling so much contentment and love to be able to run around the track on that sunny, spring day.

After the race was over, it was time to go home. The season was over, my freshman year was complete, and summer of 2014 was upon us. I was sad to be leaving college and my friends and teammates. My parents smiled as they drove me home and reminded me how homesick I was in the beginning. Gone were those days. I couldn't wait to return in the fall of next year and do it all over again.

A Summer I'll Never Forget

It was summertime and I was at my grandparents cabin swimming in the lake while Grandma sat at the end of the dock. Grandma would often come out and watch me swim. As a little girl, she'd sit there patiently as I would swim under water then jump up excitedly and ask her if I looked like a real mermaid. On this day, we smiled and chatted as I treaded water and poked my toes out into the air. Grandpa always swam this way and I could never figure out how he made it look so easy. It was harder than it looked. I explained to her how the steeplechase works and told her about my adventures from freshman year. She smiled and told me to not overwork myself. I was kind of known for that growing up. If I said I were going to do something, I put my head down and worked really hard until I accomplished it. I was a perfectionist with obsessive-compulsive behavior.

During this time in my life, my grandparents lived at the cabin in the summer and in the winter they would live in a one-story house about a half hour from the lake. Most days you could find Grandma gardening or baking while Grandpa was busy doing yard work, fixing something, or helping one of the neighbors. He was always busy. But no matter what they had going on, they often ended the night sitting on the patio watching the sunset.

The cabin has the most perfect view of the sunset. It never gets old watching the orange and purple colors as the sun sinks behind the trees. I looked up to my grandparents and felt safe in their company. This was my home away from home.

Almost every other night, Grandpa would serve up ice cream cones after dinner. Grandpa loved dessert and sometimes would eat it before his meal so he had "enough room." On the evenings we'd be sitting on the patio and Grandpa scooped the ice cream into the sugared cones, he would ask, "What flavor would everyone like? We have a lot of choices! There is vanilla, plain, regular, and white." Of course, Grandpa only had one flavor–vanilla. But that's just how he was. I love that memory of my grandpa. Sometimes I even have ice cream before dinner, and I think of him and can't help but smile. That side of the family is known for having a sweet tooth.

Until I was about twelve years old, he and my grandma lived at the cabin year-round and some of my favorite memories when I was little were Christmases at the lake. Grandma would decorate so beautifully, and the cabin always smelled of cookies. When Ann was old enough, we would spend our days ice skating, listening to Christmas music, and building a snowman on the front patio. Grandpa always played outside with us kids. Grandma and Grandpa made Christmas magical up north.

In 2014, I was living with them just through the summer. I would work at the local restaurant, waitressing at night, and I would be swimming, hanging out with my family, and running during the day. I never ended up sharing with my Grandma or Grandpa about what had happened to me in high school. My parents thought it would only worry them, and, looking back, I am happy I kept it to myself.

I viewed my past experience as an unfortunate event. Mainly, I blocked it out. I told myself I would never take for granted the good days again. I made a point to stop and just be. I never understood what a gift it is to be able to just sit in a chair and think about nothing and feel at peace. It was an amazing feeling to not have the "darkness" living in my shadows.

Kylie and Kaitlyn visited this summer. I always looked forward to the one weekend of every summer when they would come. We swam and pulled each other tubing and skiing. We had to get our traditional picture at the end of the dock of us all holding hands and jumping into the water. We sat around the bonfire and made smores and talked about our personal experiences of our freshman year apart. We laughed until we cried. I was truly happy and it felt like everything that had happened in my senior year of high school was in the rearview mirror and not a part of me anymore.

Running felt like old days, and I was eating healthy. Gone were my toxic thoughts around food. Food was energy and I listened to my body when I wanted to eat. I didn't count calories anymore and hadn't since high school. I was still underweight for my body type but I didn't obsess or try to control my food.

I ran the same road everyday and never grew tired of it. I'd been running up and down the road since I was twelve. My feet had thousands of miles on them. The first half of my run follows the shore line where I often pass many families and small children playing in the water and enjoying the summer weather. In the second portion of my run, I am engulfed in tall, beautiful pine trees. It almost feels magical. I never ran with music, so I could listen to nature and just get lost in my own thoughts.

My parents and Ann would visit in between Ann's basketball tournaments, and we'd all sit outside and play cards or play bags or croquet in the front yard. My mom is pretty competitive so it was always fun to challenge her and take her down in a game of bags.

I would go home here and there to see Dr. Anderson. As summertime went on he was amazed at my progress. He sat me and my parents down one visit and told us that I was on such a low dose of medication and was passing all my tests with flying colors. If I wanted to try and go off of medication completely, that would be an option. I looked at my parents and back at Dr. Anderson. He said some people only experience one psychotic break in their lifetime while others have to be on medication their entire life in order to avoid a relapse. He didn't know if this depression and psychosis was something that was going to be with me my whole life. We listened to his advice, and we all agreed I would try to go off medication while staying closely monitored.

Looking back on everything, I can not believe a psychiatrist, with as much history as he had, would ever suggest this. I put my full trust in this man and believed him when he said I could be a rare case.

I am not trying to paint him in a bad light. He did a lot for me and he tried his best. If it weren't for him, I would not be where I am today.

Overflowing Joy

I was off medication. I was thriving and made a promise to myself I would never let myself sink as low as I had in the past. I was excited to head back to college and see my friends and teammates. Most of all, I was determined to prove how good of a runner I truly was.

I arrived at school and unpacked my things in the new apartments on campus. Taylor and I were going to be living together! We also had two other roommates we were pretty close with. Our apartment had two bedrooms, a large living space, and a kitchen with bar stools lining the counter top. Taylor and I would be sharing one of the rooms. Taylor decided not to run on the team this year so Anna, who was also on the team, and I were the only ones in the apartment early that August.

I showed up to practice the first day and gave everyone a hug. We welcomed the incoming freshman. Jordan was captain this season, and I was so happy to be back and running with her and the other girls on the team.

Cal said, "Hi. You seem different. You look good."

I smiled genuinely and understood what he meant. I felt different. I was much more outgoing than freshman year and I felt more confident. My other teammates noticed it right away too. As the season took off, it was evident my running had improved. I was the number four runner on the team and was running with a very talented group of women. Feeling more connected to them, I mostly would hang out with the older, more mature girls. Cal seemed bemused by my confidence and better race times and seemed to take greater interest in me when it came to my running performance. I truly enjoyed every practice and every race that fall.

I wrote my running goals on a notecard and taped it to my desk. Each day I would revisit them and throughout the season I would cross one accomplishment off after another. I was very driven. I knew what I wanted to accomplish in the classroom and on the racing course.

Each day I would make a point to remember what I was grateful for. I would remind myself that life was a gift. Life and nothing in it were promised. I think deep down I knew the scariness of what happened my senior year, it still lived inside me. I tried not to think about it, but I subconsciously knew the darkness would return. I'm not sure how I had this sense.

Within the first few weeks of getting there I was having trouble sleeping. It wasn't like before; there were no bad thoughts. I was just so wide awake and had endless energy. I shared with one of my teammates that I would wake up most mornings by four in the morning and could not get myself to go back to bed. I felt so excited to start my day. I told her I was happy I was becoming a morning person, but I wanted to make sure I was getting adequate sleep. She introduced me to melatonin–a short term dietary supplement that treats insomnia. I bought a bottle at Target and began to take a pill every night before I went to bed. Even with melatonin, I was up and out of bed by 6:00 a.m. everyday. I would quietly go into the bathroom, shower, dress, straighten my hair, do my makeup, and head to the living room to do homework or read a book, sometimes stretch or do ab exercises. I would make my own coffee for my first class and eat a healthy breakfast. Some days I would even go on a bike ride before my 8 a.m. class just to soak in the fresh fall air. I would be in class intent and ready to learn at least five minutes before class started. I had chosen a major in Public Health. I decided I wanted to help the community and others around topics of preventative health and wellness. I made the Dean's list that semester.

There would be a day here or there where I would become so overwhelmed with emotions that I didn't know what to do but cry. It was as if all the happiness and energy would become so intense to the point where it was too much. I would lay on the floor in our room when Taylor wasn't home and call my dad and talk to him. I would cry and tell him I didn't know why I was crying, but I just needed to talk to someone. I promised him I wasn't sad. We would have good conversations, and he always made me feel like I wasn't crazy.

These feelings I had were different than I had ever experienced. Even during freshman year track season, when I was decreasing my medication, I never felt this kind of euphoria.

Life felt really good. I would step outside and smile and tell myself the reason I felt so much joy was because I wasn't taking life for granted anymore. It was easy to make friends and be social. My coach even had me give tours of the campus to prospective new runners for next year. He wanted me to share with them how I overcame my homesickness my first year and how I was navigating college life and running successfully.

I became close with Emily, another girl on our team who lived across the hall. We had a lot of fun together. We would often do our runs together on the weekends and paint canvases when we didn't have school work. She opened up to me at one point and told me she's dealt with mild depression. She explained her symptoms and how she coped. I listened intently to her and realized my experience only had a few similarities to her. She didn't have hallucinations or delusions, yet my diagnosis was only "major depressive illness." I didn't like that there was no explanation for all of the horror and embarrassment I went through. I pushed those thoughts aside.

Before races a group of us would get ready in our hotel room. We had matching purple ribbons we'd put in our pony tails, and we always wore a warrior tattoo on our cheek or outer thigh. Our mascot was a warrior. Each of us would write something on our hand or wrist with a sharpie so when the race got hard we could look at it, and it would give us the strength we needed to push through. I wasn't scared of the pain of running. My legs were light. In the middle of the race when my lungs would burn and my legs grew tired, I would look down at my wrist and see the word *Strength*. I would remember all I had been through in this life and how hard I worked to be where I was. I would think about God's strength. I would always remind myself that I was not guaranteed to be here. Running is a gift, and I was so grateful to be able to compete. That was all I needed in those moments.

After the regional meet had ended, we waited as a team to hear the final results. It felt like forever, but they finally announced our team had qualified for the DII National Championships. At that moment I became overwhelmed with emotions. Senior year and Georgia and Johnson all flashed through my mind, and I could not believe where I had been and where I was standing now. I remember looking at my parents and breaking down into tears of happiness. They smiled, and my dad got teary eyed. They knew how much this meant to me.

Our team raced on December 6th in Louisville, KY in the national championship race. It had rained for three days straight leading up to the race and the course was wet and muddy. We were all covered from head to toe by the time the race had ended. It was the most fun I'd ever had in a race.I didn't know it then but this would be the last competitive cross country meet I would ever participate in.

Four days after Nationals, eight other women from my cross country team and I boarded a flight to Ahuahu, Hawaii. We had planned this trip over the summer. One of the girl's parents owned a house inland from Honolulu, and the team was invited to come and stay as long as we paid for our plane tickets, food, and excursions. It was an opportunity I couldn't pass up. It was an amazing experience. Hawaii is one of the most beautiful places I have ever seen. Fornine days, my friends and I visited every side of the island. We swam in the ocean, took surfing lessons, hiked to breathtaking lookouts, saw gorgeous waterfalls, and experienced the local culture. It looked so odd seeing holiday lights and hearing Christmas music throughout the tropical island during our time there; we were all used to a cold, white Christmas at home in Minnesota. We were told by our coach to have fun and only run twenty to twenty-five minutes every other day to give our legs a break.

Running on Empty

While I was in Hawaii, my behavior began to change ever so slightly. I became more sensitive and irritated. I didn't want to gain weight and I was worried I would lose all of the progress I had made throughout the season. On the runs we'd do as a team, I'd always add on an extra five to ten minutes even though the captains encouraged me not to. I was doing abs in the mornings and began to restrict my food again.

I arrived home just before Christmas day. I was home for a week or two. The desire to push myself harder with my training continued. I was outside doing workouts even on days as cold as five degrees. I was very critical of myself and there were times when I would explode with frustration at my parents or Ann for things that would normally never phase me. There were no intrusive thoughts, just an obsession around controlling my food and exercise.

In January, I was back at school ready for the indoor track season to begin. The team had an overarching head coach, but Cal was the distance coach. Back were the days of restricting and purging. Taylor and I had grown really close earlier in the year. She told me I needed to be eating more food, and she told me to stop weighing myself. But I was in denial and didn't want to listen to her. I know now that my obsessive-compulsive tendencies seem to spike when I am experiencing severe changes in mood.

I also became very obsessive and compulsive with my training to the point where it became extremely unhealthy and unsustainable. I tried my best to come across as confident even when I felt confused. I lost my appetite like I had in 2013. I couldn't gauge how much to eat because there was no desire. Then the paranoia returned. When I was walking through campus I had the sense that someone was following me. I shook it off and told myself it was all in my head. I remember standing in the kitchen of my apartment eating a snack and listening to the movie Taylor was watching. For a split second I thought the television was talking about me. I knew I was close to losing touch with reality again and I needed to get home ASAP before my world came crashing down on me. I called my parents, and we made an appointment with Dr. Anderson for Friday, the next day. I had only been off medication for six months.

I called Kylie and told her what was happening. She was calm this time and told me everything would be all right. She told me to be honest with the doctors.

I went to tell Cal I needed to go home for a weekend and would be back on Sunday. He asked if everything was okay. I broke down into sobs in his office.

I told him, "I don't understand what is wrong with me. No one understands."

He looked at me with shock and concern. I immediately got embarrassed by my outburst and hurried out of his office.

Floating Kites

I walked into the psychiatric clinic that Friday. As I sat in the waiting room with my parents, I felt like I had a pit in my stomach as I waited for what was coming. I excused myself to the bathroom and began to sob. I didn't want to be back with Dr. Edwardson or in any psychiatric clinic. I didn't want to be like all the other people in the waiting room. I didn't want to lose myself again or feel the terrible pain return. I wiped my eyes, looked into the mirror, and whispered to myself, "It's going to be okay. You are so strong and you've done this before." I went back into the waiting room, sat with my mom and dad and waited until it was time for my appointment.

Dr. Anderson called us into his office. He told me I looked good, I seemed good. I began to cry and told him something was terribly wrong. I told him I felt like Wile E. Coyote, the character from Looney Toons. I described the scene where he was running so fast and couldn't stop, until he fell off a cliff. I meant that I was going to lose touch with reality again. My brain was causing me to get confused again, and I didn't know how to slow it down. I was going to crash. He decided to put me back on Risperidone. I was to take my first dose that night.

He asked when was the last time my period had been. At the age of twenty, I had not had my period in over eighteen months. I looked at it as a good thing. I liked that I didn't have to deal with cramps or bloating. At the time, I was even proud it was missing because it meant I was a true athlete and I was working hard. He prescribed me birth control in order to regulate my hormones. He said this might help stabilize my mood.

Having a period is healthy and natural. I abused my body in late high school and early college. My body has done amazing things, but we all only get one of them. I wish I had taken better care of my younger self. In high school and college I didn't think of the consequences of being underweight and not addressing the absence of my menstrual cycle. When I was finally given a proper diagnosis, put on medication, and stabilized, my disordered eating ceased to exist. I am now at a very natural and healthy weight and have thankfully gained back a natural monthly cycle.

I stared at the little yellow pill of Risperidone that night knowing what side effects were going to hit me once I began to take this regularly again. I reluctantly swallowed it. Moments after, I became overwhelmed with anxiety and akathisia—the sense of restlessness and intense need to move. It is one of the most uncomfortable feelings I have ever felt.

Ann had a basketball game that night, and my parents asked me to come with them to the game so I wouldn't be home alone. Sue was there to watch Ann play and I gave her a big hug. I sat uncomfortably in the stands. The entire time I was either so drowsy that I couldn't keep my eyes open or I had the temptation to move around and pace. At halftime I walked out to the hallway. No matter how much I walked back and forth, the urge to move would not go away. I would not wish this feeling upon anyone. These feelings persisted through the night and into Saturday.

Saturday night I was home, lying on the couch and watching a movie with my family. I became more anxious and the feeling of akathisia was not subsiding. As I lay on the couch, I felt like I was outside of my body staring down at myself. I told my parents I was going to lie down upstairs in my room. I went upstairs and curled up on my bed still feeling strange and uncomfortable. I closed my eyes. When I opened them I saw kites floating above my head, bobbing against the ceiling of my room. I knew it was a hallucination. I squeezed my eyes shut again and told myself they weren't real, I was imagining them. I opened my eyes again and they were still there in the same spot. At this point my dad walked into my room to check on me. He suddenly had tattoos on his face of skulls and scary outlines. I couldn't answer him. It was like I lost my ability to speak.

I didn't know it at the time, but I was experiencing a symptom of psychosis called alogia or "poverty of speech."

My parents knew I was not well. They told me we were going to go to the hospital. I got in the car, and soon after we pulled into the emergency room at Johnson Hospital.

An Accurate Diagnosis

I sat down in a room and a nurse and doctor came in. The nurse took my vitals and the doctor asked why I was there. I still couldn't speak. I was filled with anger and rage. I am not an angry person so this was out of character for me. I imagined myself punching the nurse in the face but held back the temptation and finally told her I needed help.

"I am seeing things that aren't real."

She asked if I felt like hurting myself.

I answered honestly, "No."

She made the decision to admit me to the inpatient psychiatric unit where I had been only two years prior. I changed into a hospital gown and waited in the emergency room until a room and bed became available for me.

For two days I waited and I slept in a hospital bed behind a curtain in the ER. My parents and Ann visited me each day. Ann thought the hospital socks were cool—the red and blue wool ones they give to patients. We would sit on the edge of my bed dangling our feet in our matching hospital socks.

My hallucinations were gone, but I felt like I had hit a wall. I was still somewhat confused and extremely exhausted. My brain felt broken. My mom gave me a set of clothes and my school work.

I called the administration office at my college and told them I was in the hospital and didn't know when I would be back. They said they would let my professors know and I could work with them when I got back to school in order to make up for my missed work. I also called Cal and told him I was in the hospital for mental health reasons and I would do what I could to return to school. He told me not to worry and take care of myself.

While I was in the ER, I slept, ate, did school work, and walked laps around the nurses station so as to not gain weight. Finally a bed opened up for me. I had been through this before. I was prepared and determined to work hard and get out as soon as possible so I could return to school to continue to run and pursue my degree. I did not want to get behind on anything or have to stay in school for an extra semester. As I reflect on this, it wouldn't have been so bad if I had taken some time off to recover. I wish I wouldn't have been so hard on myself. Constantly pushing myself out of my comfort zone was my way of life for twenty years. In the hospital, I refused to give myself any time to relax and just be. This was a mistake. I should have been nicer to myself and made my health my top priority. I was letting my productivity define me. School would have still been there when I was ready. My friends would have still been there. If you're having a bad day, mentally, I hope you set your outward priorities aside and treat it like you have an actual physical health injury. My grandma always says, "If you have your health and your family, you have everything," and I truly believe that.

Each day I would attend group therapy, see my doctor, and do my school work with the books I had. I also began to journal again for the first time since winter of 2014. I wanted to track my feelings and emotions each day.

When I met with my doctor at one point, he told me he had never met a patient who had had a psychotic break and days later was doing advanced anatomy homework. He said I was a rare case, and he could see my determination to be released. He asked about my weight. I was at the lowest weight I had ever been. I told him that I believed if I were skinnier, I would be happier. He asked if that was working for me. I looked down at my lap and shook my head "No." He said he highly recommends seeing a therapist about my eating habits and about my mental illness when I am discharged.

I made cookies for all the patients and nurses one day. I sat them out on the tables for others to take as they pleased. As I sat doing school work, I heard a nurse comment, "I bet whoever made these is trying to poison us." I instantly became irritated. This nurse who was here to help all of these patients, including myself, was stereotyping us. I could not believe what he said. I approached him and told him that I had made the cookies. He looked down, embarrassed that I had heard him. I walked away.

Each day I would do my makeup and braid my hair in order to feel and appear put together. They even let me shave my legs one day with a two blade razor; however, a nurse had to watch me do it. I received a pass just after my second day.

One time I used the pass to go down and swim in the hospital's pool. Halfway through the week, my doctor asked if I felt comfortable taking a day pass. This meant that I would be able to go home for the day and return that night to sleep and let him know how I felt. I agreed and that day my dad picked me up. I ran, took a bath, and ate lunch and dinner with my family before heading back to the hospital.

They were still trying to determine my correct diagnosis. I looked at paint splotches with a specialist at the hospital and told him what I saw in each of them. I took a two hundred plus multiple choice test about my personality, feelings, and viewpoints on different things. I answered everything as honestly as I could. I believe it was a neuropsychology test used to help determine what type of mental illness a person has.

Finally, near the end of my one week stay, the doctor met with me and told me he thought I may have bipolar 1 disorder. I looked at him and quickly disagreed. What I had thought bipolar meant was that a person was either in a good mood and happy or acted like a bitch. I wasn't like that. He explained that that was not what it was. Bipolar disorder is a mental disorder that includes periods of elation and depression. He explained that bipolar 1 meant that it was a more severe case than bipolar 2, often with the patient experiencing at least one psychotic break. I thought about it and it made total sense.

All that time during fall semester when I thought I was extremely healthy and just overly happy, I was experiencing mania, a part of bipolar disorder which is marked by great excitement and euphoria. The way he described it was that every person experiences moods on a pole. One end of the pole is a happy mood and one end is a sad mood. I was experiencing different states of mood and energy more extremely than other people to a point where it was causing me to be unable to function.

I told him I knew of no one else in my family who had ever been diagnosed with bipolar disorder or any mental illness for that matter. I didn't understand why I would have it. He explained that most times it is genetic, but sometimes it is just a chemical imbalance in the brain and no one has an answer to why it happens. He said it was no one's fault.

He explained to me that because I was manic for such a long time, my brain could not maintain the high energy it was exerting. I would experience major depression once more. He assured me that this time I would have a good team of experts outside of the hospital helping me get through it. It may take time to stabilize my mood, but he promised I would get there. As long as I was on medication, it would be very unlikely for me to lose touch with reality. I felt relieved to finally have an answer to all that had happened to me over the last two and half years. I wasn't crazy.

I was determined I could overcome this depression. In my journal I wrote a promise to myself to never attempt suicide again. I told myself that if those intrusive thoughts ever came back and I didn't want to live, I would live for my parents, for Ann, for my family, for Kylie, and for all my other friends who loved me.

January 27th, 2015 journal entry - the day before I was discharged:

> *I refuse to give up... to give in to unhealthy temptations. I will take care of my body, feed it the right things and enough, give it enough sleep, force myself to relax and keep a positive mindset. I will accomplish what I set out to accomplish. Because if I give up, that's giving in and letting the depression win. Depression will not win. And by giving up and/or giving in, that's living by the label. I refuse to let it*

define me as a person. Depression and I are not one in the same. Depression lies, and I will never be sucked in ever again.

Screw Perfection

I was back on campus two weeks after I initially left the school. I could feel the depression, but I did my best to push it aside and get back into my routine. I thought I could go back to school and things would be the same as they were before I left, but that was not the case. How I was living my life earlier that fall was unsustainable and unrealistic, and I had an enormous amount of healing to do.

I started to see a therapist off of campus, and Dr. Anderson remained my doctor for the time being. I think he felt guilty for all that had happened because he gave me his home phone number and said I could call him night or day if I needed something and could not reach him at the office.

I dropped a couple of my classes and ended up making them up over the summer. My grades declined a bit, but all of my professors were understanding and lenient as I made up work and took their tests.

I shared a few details of the last two weeks with Taylor, and she was extremely supportive. She was taking a course on mental health in school at the time so she was pretty knowledgeable on what I was dealing with. She would cook and bake for me, encouraging me to put some natural weight back on. There would be times when I would cry uncontrollably, and she would sit with me and encourage me that I could overcome the depression. She told me I needed to be nice to myself and to not put so much pressure on myself. I am forever grateful for how much of her time she gave me when she could have been focusing on school work and her nursing clinicals.

Intrusive thoughts would come and make me feel like I wasn't good enough. I journaled all of these thoughts and feelings and shared them with my therapist, Mary. Even though I was secure in my treatment plan, I still had symptoms and had a lot of recovery to do both mentally and physically. It takes time to reach a state of balance again.

Cal told me I could come sit and do homework in his office at any point during the day, and I could train with the team without competing in any races until outdoor season began. I felt good about this plan. I wasn't quite sure how to share my diagnosis with him or my teammates. I was very ashamed of it and wanted to hide it. I didn't want to tell anyone I hallucinated or ever had thoughts about hurting myself because I wanted them to look up to me. Still, there was that never ending question, *Why had I been absent for two weeks?* I wasn't ready to share and so I acted like nothing happened. I'm sure it was confusing and awkward.

Practices were tough. The feeling of having heavy legs on my runs returned. Emily was always so sweet and let me run with her and talk about my depression. Sometimes I would just cry, and other times I would explain how constantly overwhelmed I felt. She understood me and having her be there to lean on brought me comfort.

April 4th, 2015 journal entry:

> *Sometimes I don't feel like myself. I feel completely out of it, almost hazy. I don't know what my priorities are anymore or what I want to do with myself. When I interact with people it feels forced. I am sad. I'm trying to be strong but it's like all the things I used to care about don't matter. I forced myself to run this morning but it seems like nothing can give me relief and nothing can satisfy me. All I want to do is sleep and not think about anything.*

I talked to my parents everyday. I would cry to my dad and tell him how hard it was to carry on. He would remain calm and encourage me and tell me I could do it. "One day at a time," he would say. "Don't think about the next day until tomorrow comes." It helped. I will always be thankful to my parents for all their support and listening even though they didn't quite understand exactly how I felt. I know sharing my dark feelings and pain hurt them immensely, but it meant more to them that I was being honest and open about what was going on inside of my head then just pretending to be okay. That's all they asked for. They saved my life and their support and love has gotten me to where I am today.

Every time terrible thoughts would come, I'd think of how much my family and friends needed me and open my journal to remind myself of the promise I made to myself.

Finally, the outdoor season came. I ran my first race in the 1500 meter. It felt awful. I could feel every step I took, and it was extremely difficult. When I finished the race I felt akathisia and anger wash over me all at the same time. I did my best to act normal even though I had a strong urge to move about unnaturally.

Cal approached me and said, "That's a personal best! You're back!"

Shit, I thought to myself. Yes, my times are good, and I looked fit and all, but I was still far from okay or back to my old self.

Prior to having a mental break, my world revolved around running. I wanted to keep my enthusiasm, but depression can make people lose interest in what they normally like to do, like running. I stopped caring, even though I truly wanted to care. I know Cal meant well and his job was to produce high quality athletes, but that is not what I needed to hear. It only caused more pressure that I put on myself. I should have said something but I didn't want to let him down and I didn't want him to give up on me so I did not share these feelings with him.

I ran two more races that season, both in the steeplechase. Every race I felt the same; I felt every single time my feet would touch the ground, and I had an urge to just walk off the track. After each race, I only felt anger and akathisia. It was terrible. To my immense relief, Cal told me I did not need to race anymore and he would not put me on the conference team so I could head home early and focus on rest and training over the summer.

Three days later, our head track coach sent out the roster he had submitted to the NCAA with the final names of the participants competing in the DII conference meet in only two short weeks. My name was on the list. My heart sank. I could not do it. *But my name is on the list,* I thought to myself, *I have to do it.* I visited Cal's office and asked him what had happened. He let me know that the head track coach liked my effort and performance so much during the season that he took it upon himself to add me to the roster. I'm sure the head coach thought he was doing me a favor. I felt overwhelmed with depression and all I had on my plate with finals and day-to-day life. I was struggling just to take care of myself and show up to class on time. I did not want to appear weak to Cal, so I said I would race.

From the ages of eighteen to twenty-three, I viewed my depression and all the feelings that came with it as a weakness. But it is not a matter of being strong or weak; I was sick. Plain and simple. And that is okay. It is okay to not feel good, and I should have been nicer to myself. I eventually realized I needed to stop fighting it and be kinder to myself. You can't "talk yourself out of it" or "suck it up." When people used these phrases it was extremely hurtful even though they thought they were giving me advice. I don't like the phrase "mental illness" either. I prefer "mental health injury" because that is truly what it is. My brain was injured and not producing the chemicals it needed to function normally. Like a broken leg or having diabetes, I was hurt. No one says "talk yourself out of it" to your cancer or any physical injury for that matter. Because you can't and it just doesn't work that way.

I forced myself to go to practice every day and push through my workouts. I did my best to appear confident even though I was far from it. I met with Mary and told her how much I dreaded the race coming up. I told her I was scared that if I were to run it, I would become so overwhelmed that I was going to run off the track halfway through the race and potentially hurt myself. I was at my breaking point. She told me not to go and to stop trying to be so strong because that was not what I needed in order to heal.

There was a case in 1986 where a NCAA star runner became so overwhelmed during a race she was running that she ran off the track, climbed over a fence, and threw herself head first off a 50 foot bridge. She is alive today, paralyzed from the waist down. In the *New York Times*, she was described by a friend as "a shy girl, an introvert. She seemed to put pressure on herself that she had to run fast every race." She later said she did it because she was so scared of failure. She was an extreme perfectionist.

I am so thankful Mary talked some sense into me and made me realize I didn't have to be strong or perfect. I should have put running higher than everything else. My priorities were off.

Two days before the bus was set to leave, I went to see Cal to tell him I could not run in the meet. He did not take this well. He looked at it as lost points for our overall team score. I felt like a failure but my mind was made up. I did not want to end up like the NCAA star from 1986. I left the conversation feeling confident with my decision but defeated and at the same time, the depression loomed over me. I headed home for the summer and wouldn't talk to Cal again for two months.

May 5th, 2015 journal entry:

> *Yesterday was not a very good day. I told Cal I could not go to the conference. He was angry. This is my decision for me. And yes, I took someone else's spot, lost points for the team, and I didn't follow through. But I just really need to go home. I got together with some teammates afterwards, and they said they were proud of me for doing what I needed to do. I am so scared of feeling the way I do after I run hard. When I feel that way I am frightened I'm going to act unnatural and out of control. I don't want anyone to see me that way. I didn't mean to hurt Cal or others on the team by not going. This summer I really need to figure some stuff out and focus on myself.*

Life is not always about running. And sometimes things get scary because you aren't sure what's gonna happen next, but really, there's no need to be scared or doubt anything because God has a plan—a plan better than anything we could sketch up ourselves.

One Day at a Time

It was summertime in 2015, just a month after I walked away from the opportunity to perform in the conference meet. The depression was still intense. I was living at the cabin again, but due to my grandparent's health they came out less often. I had family who stayed in the cabin with me once in a while and a few relatives that lived close by. I surrounded myself with them in order to distract myself from my pain.

My parents still hadn't shared my story with any of my extended family members. Only my aunt and uncle who lived in Minneapolis were aware since John had been there with me during my time at Cherish. At first, I thought my parents were not sharing my diagnosis and struggles with my family because they were ashamed of me, but I was wrong. They wanted to protect me and allow me to tell those I trusted when I felt comfortable. It was my story, not just theirs. I am so grateful they let me choose what I wanted to share and who I wanted to share it with when I felt ready.

I met with Mary through virtual meetings once in a while to share with her how I was doing. I would journal every single day.

Getting through the day was a struggle. My shifts at the restaurant began at 3:30 p.m. I would often sleep until ten or eleven, eat, do some online class work, run if I could get myself out the door, and either nap in bed or on the beach until it was time to go to work.

Some days I would crawl to the bathroom just to take a shower. My severe depression made it a very sad summer, but I did my best.

June 6th, 2015 journal entry:

> *I've come to realize I set these strict rules for myself (restricting food, running farther and faster) that I can't keep up with myself. I get obsessed. I have a belief that the more I do—the better I'll feel—the happier I'll be. And that's not always true. I don't want to live like that anymore because it sucks the fun out of things and makes me feel like I have to be perfect and the best. When I do this I put pressure on myself that is too intense and unattainable. I had a breakthrough moment when I laid down for a nap today. I realized running does not need to control my life. I don't have to be on the team next year if it's going to be too much. I think it'd be cool to get more involved in my major, join clubs, and find an identity in something other than running. Why do I put so much pressure on myself to be this "star athlete"? Really, no one cares and it's kind of sad if that's what my main focus is.*

July hit and I made a difficult decision. I called Cal and let him know I was going to quit the team. He was understanding and when I spoke to some of the women who stayed on the team the next couple years, they described him as being more open and willing to learn when runners on the team were dealing with mental health hurdles such as eating disorders, anxiety, and depression. I like to think I played a role in that. We ended up connecting again after I graduated. At this point I shared some of my story with him, and we now stay in touch. He never did apologize for what had happened during my last track season on the team.

I was experiencing such intense depression that it was impossible for me to get adequate training in which was needed in order to continue on the team. I remember laying on the couch in the cabin, crying to my parents. "I'm not a runner anymore, I'm nothing. I don't know who I am at all and I feel like a failure."

Often, college students who are done competing experience loss of identity and, for me, the depression intensified these feelings. It is really common to feel lost after leaving a sport, and it's not something many people talk about. Running was my life for over nine years, and I didn't know who I was or what I was going to do with my time.

August 18th, 2015 journal entry:

> *It's been days since I last made an entry. I haven't felt like writing anything lately because life has been tough. When I say tough I mean that I feel like I'm not living. It feels as if I'm in a clear bubble watching everyone live life, going about their day...and I'm just there... But I'm not because I can't feel joy from the activity I am doing. I can't smell the warm summer air and feel at peace. I can't go get something done because it feels like the hardest challenge in the entire world and if I can peel myself off my bed to go do it, what's the point? The other day I was in the cabin at the lake feeling this way and it scared me that I won't be able to go back to school if I'm sick like this. Because after dealing with this for two years on and off I've learned that no matter how much you push yourself and wear a painted smile on your face, you can not beat it. Not without help and medication and doctors. So that is the plan. I've increased my medication. I will live— actually live.*

For nine entire months I remained depressed. Living like that was the hardest thing I've ever done in my life, hands down. If I had to do it again, I'd be terrified. But I would because life is worth living, and I don't believe God would put me through anything I can't handle.

Eventually, I was put on all new medication. It was life changing and had very few side effects. Finally the depression began to lift.

One thing that's difficult with a new mental health diagnosis is that there is no right answer to what the treatment plan should be when it comes to medication, and oftentimes, it can take two to four weeks just for the medication to take any effect. It is a difficult process and a waiting game as doctors try new prescription methods.

Everyone is different; what works for me may not be the right fit for you and that's okay! If you are someone who is taking medication for the first time, please be patient and know it can take a bit to find something that helps you. Also, read up on what you are taking and putting in your body. You do get a say based on what the side effects look like and what you feel comfortable with. Life is so beautiful and worth it and relief will come. Sometimes it just takes patience and trust in your doctors and the other health professionals you are working with.

I gained over twenty pounds. Although I hated it, it is what my body needed. I finally had my period back. Walking away from the team was the best decision in so many ways, even though I didn't see it right away. It forced me to be less critical of myself over time, focus on food less, and find interests in things I didn't have time for when I was on the team. It helped me find balance. I didn't need to be running fifty miles a week anymore. I became kinder to my body.

I stayed close with Taylor, Emily, Jordan, and a few others through and past college. I learned that some teammates are lifelong friends and some are just teammates, and that is okay. I was a bridesmaid in one of their weddings after college and it felt so special to stand next to my dear friend. I tried to find friends outside of the sport but in all honesty, I didn't form any strong friendships my junior or senior year of college.

My last two years of college had severe ups and downs. There were good times and bad times. I had nothing close to a normal college experience, but, then again, what is normal? My hard work and determination allowed me to graduate on time.

There would be times where I would see something or smell something that would remind me of spring break or Cherish, and I would panic and sometimes hyperventilate. For example, I joined a new gym after college where the towels at the gym smelt strongly of bleach. I had not faced or accepted the trauma I had experienced. You cannot move on unless you face the pain of your past, and I was scared to do this because I knew it would be difficult and painful.

I struggled with stigma and self confidence. I shared pieces of my story with very few people and believed I would never find true love because no one would accept me if they knew what I had done and believed about myself at times in my life. I still viewed myself as inadequate for having a mental illness. If you have a mental illness, know it only defines you if you let it. It took me a while, but eventually my confidence grew back. I HAVE bipolar, I AM NOT bipolar.

A Broken Proposal

Near the end of my time at school, I met a man who would later become my boyfriend. Out of respect for him, I will call him Joe. He hung out with Taylor, myself, and some other friends beginning in the spring of my junior year. He was nice, but I only viewed him as a friend.

One day when we were hanging out, he opened up to me and told me that sometimes he deals with anxiety. I gave him some advice and also shared with him that I had some mental health struggles myself. He was kind and wanted to know more. I opened up to him and shared my story without going into too much detail. I cried as I spoke about my experiences and my diagnosis with bipolar disorder, and, when I finished, I held my breath as I waited to hear what he would say. Surprisingly, he did not pass any judgment. He told me it was okay and that everyone deals with a challenge in their life and it was nothing to be ashamed of. I couldn't believe he didn't view me as crazy or a monster.

I didn't look at him in a romantic way at the time, but I told myself this might be the only man who would accept me for what I was. We began to date.

He was my boyfriend for a little over two years and I had a pretty good time with him. He was extremely nice to me and I could tell he genuinely loved me. We did a lot together but had little in common. He didn't love the outdoors or physical activity as much as I did. He was the first serious relationship I ever had and I told myself I could mold him into what I wanted in a boyfriend. He would often tell me he was set on marrying me one day, and I went along with it.

I went to a wedding in the early spring of 2018. As I sat in the audience I watched as the couple in front of me recited their vows. I saw the way they looked at each other with pure love and respect. I realized at this moment I could never look at Joe in that way. No matter how hard I wanted to love him the way he loved me, there would be no way I could stand at an altar, look him in the eye, and share feelings with him that just weren't there. At this point I should have broken it off because it would've saved a lot of hurt feelings and heartbreak, but we ended up dating for three more months after that.

I had an idea he could be thinking about proposing, and I still stayed with him. I feel terrible for leading him on, using him, and I should have known better. I had convinced myself no one would ever love me like he did, and, therefore, I held on longer than I should have. He ended up proposing and my heart sank because I knew it wasn't right. I didn't love him, and I am truly sorry I caused him so much pain. I said "Yes" not knowing what to do, and we were engaged for a few weeks before I eventually broke it off.

During the short time we were engaged, I ran a 5k in Minneapolis. As I ran, the stress about my engagement felt overwhelming. All of a sudden I just stopped running and a calm washed over me. I heard a voice in my head say, "You don't have to marry him and that's okay. It will be okay."

In this moment I found the courage to do what I needed to do, to do what was right.

A couple days after my 5k, I broke Joe's heart. After I left the relationship, I felt so much relief and improved confidence. I even felt happier. A weight which had been there for months was lifted. I saved us both a lot of hurt and unhappiness which would have come had I married him and forced something that wasn't there. I told myself I would not settle for a relationship my heart was not fully invested in.

My Time with Grandpa

Around the time I graduated college, my grandma became ill and had to stay in the hospital for about a month. My grandparents were still living in their one-story house during this time, and my grandpa could not be left alone because he was in the early stages of dementia. I did not have a job at this point and anxiously volunteered to go live with him to help take care of him.

No matter how confused he became in the last few years of his life, he never had a bad attitude about it. He was always such a positive person my entire life, and I never heard him speak badly about other people, even if he did not agree with them. He worked extremely hard to make a good life for himself and his family.

I looked up to him immensely and wanted to be just like him. I would ask him what his favorite season was and he told me all of them; he had no favorite because they all brought something unique and special. I wanted to have this viewpoint and not fear fall and wintertime.

We would do puzzles or play cards and he would pretend he didn't know how to play the game we were playing, often joking about his dementia, and then end up winning because he was so smart and such a trickster. We would laugh and talk for hours.

It never bothered me that he would retell the same stories multiple times. I cherished every moment and was just so thankful I had him all to myself. He was my best friend and my hero and often referred to me as "Grandpa's girl." He would always tell me he was so proud of the young woman I was becoming.

One day as we sat out on the patio, looking out at the pond, I asked, "Grandpa, how come you're always so happy?"

I thought about how unfair it was that he had to deal with dementia and slowly lose his memory. He was also in a wheelchair at this point in his life. He had been such an active man his entire life, and now he was dependent on his chair. He looked at me and smiled, with a twinkle in his eye.

"Happiness is a choice," he said. "Life is not always easy, but it is what you make of it, and I choose happiness."

I decided at this moment I would do my best to live this way. Even in my depressive episodes, I could choose to always have a positive outlook on life.

At the age of eighty years old he told me that sometimes he felt like he was still nineteen even though his body had aged. He told me that age is just a number.

My grandpa passed away in the spring of 2020. I was with him in his last days and held his hand. Although it was extremely sad, it was so special that he was surrounded by his family when he left this world. I still talk to him almost everyday and tell him how I'm doing and remind him how much I love him and look up to him. I let him know I am extremely proud to be his granddaughter. I don't know if he gets my messages, but I truly believe he is in a better place and that makes me happy. I'm reminded of him when I'm at the cabin—our special place. And I see him in my dad, his children, and sometimes even in myself.

Healing

I changed doctors a couple times in order to find someone who was a good fit for me. Dr. Anderson did not know enough about Latuda to feel comfortable with adjusting the dose because it was such a new drug that would not become generic until at least eight years after I began taking it. This made it extremely expensive and not covered by most insurance companies.

I had to be selective of where I would work based on the type of insurance they offered so I could afford my medication. I wanted to have a plan and be prepared if I ever had to stay inpatient again. I eventually found a job at a startup company that partially covered my medication and had pretty decent coverage. My new doctor would give me samples of Latuda throughout the year since it was outrageously priced. I eventually was able to use coupons that would help me to supplement the remaining cost.

My moods are affected by the change in season and major life changes. I had ups and downs that always seemed to happen around the same time of year. I often experience mania in the fall and sometimes I would experience depression in winter and early spring. This cycle would continue from 2014 until today. However, it's gotten much more mild as the years pass by and sometimes doesn't happen at all. I feared fall because I knew it would affect my stability and disrupt my lifestyle, but I remembered that Grandpa viewed every season as a blessing and I wanted to get to that point.

In 2018, I met my current therapist, Richard. I had tried a handful of therapists since I graduated and wasn't able to see Mary anymore since I no longer lived in my college town. There was no one I related to or trusted. I told myself this was the last therapist I would try and if it didn't work, I just would go without seeing anyone. My advice to anyone looking for a therapist is to be patient and don't give up. Today I am leaps and bounds ahead of where I would be if I had not found a therapist I could trust. Sometimes it takes time to find a therapist you feel connected to. Before I met with Richard, my previous therapist told me I did wrong by graduating in four years and should have taken time off from school. She may have had a point, but I am proud of how hard I worked. I want a therapist who builds me up, not someone who tears me down.

That summer day, I sat in Richard's office with a bleak mindset. He asked me why I was there, so I told him that I have bipolar 1 disorder and I was told seeing a therapist would improve my quality of life. We vibed right from the beginning. I really appreciated how he would let me lead the conversations and he never asked too many questions or pressed me for information I was not ready to share. I felt comfortable in his presence and he slowly gained my trust.

September 2018 journal entry

> *I am thinking about telling my therapist the extensive details about my senior year of high school. The thought brings so much pain. I went through hell for the longest time and I completely blocked it out. I want it to never have happened. I can only imagine what my therapist will think. I was insane and psychotic and awful. How I survived the pain and embarrassment I don't know. How crazy is it that I graduated in four years and have a good job after all that? These memories make me feel so much shame. I lost the ability to think clearly, to love, sleep, remember, to feel. When I did feel it felt like a toothache—but my entire body. No amount of external love, prayer, or exercise could save me. I hate remembering. I hate that I went through that. For a long time I hated myself. But now and always I want to help myself. I want to not be ashamed.*

After about three months of seeing him, I decided it was time to do the really hard thing and share with him my psychotic breaks. He was the first professional I told my story to in extensive detail. I trusted him and we had formed a good relationship, one I never felt with my other therapists. I sat down in his office that fall and I told him I wanted to talk to him about something. He didn't say anything and waited for me to continue. Just the thought of sharing my past made me break into tears. I covered my face because I felt embarrassed for him to see me be so emotional. I finally lowered my hands and began to share my story, starting from the winter of 2013. I told him everything. I told him about senior year, about spring break, about Cherish and Johnson and my suicide attempt. I then shared my relapse that happened in college. I went into every detail, leaving nothing out, no matter how embarrassing it was. I intentionally didn't make eye contact with him as I relived my painful past. I felt so much shame and was scared of how he would react. He sat calmly as I let everything out. It was painful, but after I finished I felt so much relief.

I carried around shame, trauma, fear, and a story I trusted no one with for over five years. I have to admit, once I let go of all that hurt, I experienced a few days of anxiety and stress, but it eventually got better. Richard described it as "ripping off a bandaid." All that time I thought I was protecting myself by suppressing my memory and pretending like the shame and pain weren't there. I carried around all my baggage like an open wound. By facing my past and all my fears, I took the first step in my healing process. Richard helped me through it every step of the way. There are still times today where I'll remember something painful from my past or go through a depressive episode, and we meet and talk through it.

October 8th, 2018 journal entry:

> *Feelings of shame are slowly subsiding. I am trying to not be too hard on myself. What happened to me was not my fault. I want to be okay and not embarrassed. This illness is really serious, disabling and for some people - lethal. I feel so fortunate to have such a strong support system and loving family. I am strong, hard working, caring and compassionate—more so now than before my very first episode. I don't wish anyone to experience anywhere near the amount terror and pain that I experienced. But like Richard said, it has made me stronger and shaped me into the person I am today. I want to be the best version of myself. I also don't want to be scared of my illness.*

When I have an off day or a really good day, I journal about it in detail and leave nothing out. Almost every day I write down five things I am grateful for. Not only do I write them down, but I take the time to feel gratitude. Sometimes it's as simple as the smell of coffee or a cloudless sky, but it helps me see the beauty in the little things. Today when I smell bleach, I think about the hospital in Georgia and my experiences there, but there is no more pain, sadness, or fear. I just think about it, accept it, then let it go.

If it weren't for Richard, I would not be able to share my story with you at this time because I never would have been ready. He taught me that people can either choose to live in love or fear. For a long time I lived in fear. I feared failure, I feared I wasn't good enough, I feared what others thought about me, I feared I was unlovable, I feared myself. That is not the way I want to live my life. I choose love, and as you read about my story, I hope you choose love too.

How I Cope

I learned how to meditate from my therapist as well. It seems simple, sitting and focusing on just your breath, but it took me a lot of practice, and I am still working on mastering the skill. If I'm meditating correctly, I am focusing on my breath, not the past or future, just that very moment. It clears my mind and I just sit in a positive state of being. It works when I am having a bad day and washes all my intrusive thoughts and overwhelming feelings away.

I found ways to cope and a routine I am able to maintain to be stable and my best self. Below are things that have worked for me and helped me to stay on track to live a successful life:

- ⊙ Recording my feelings in my journal so I can look back on good memories and past episodes in order to learn from them.
- ⊙ Interrupting my negative and intrusive thoughts with positive mantras to shift my thinking.
- ⊙ Implementing uplifting distractions when I am feeling down such as listening to music, playing with my dogs, watching funny movies, spending time with the people I love, etc.
- ⊙ Exercising and moving my body—in moderation. I don't run more than twenty miles a week and have found joy in exercise outside of running.
- ⊙ Being open to sharing with my loved ones ways they can help me.
- ⊙ Staying on a schedule. I go to bed at the same time every night and do my best to not oversleep.
- ⊙ Going to therapy, seeing a psychiatrist, and never missing a dose of my medication even if I feel like I don't need to take it.

- ⊙ Not abusing drugs or alcohol.
- ⊙ Nourishing my body with healthy foods.
- ⊙ Meditating for ten minutes a day.
- ⊙ Always having something on the calendar to look forward to.
- ⊙ Being nice to myself and treating myself with respect. I often remind myself I am doing the best I can.

I have reconnected with old friends who have influenced me throughout my life and shared with them how much of an impact they had on me, even if they didn't know it at the time. It has been so relieving to be able to know I can speak openly with my friends and family about my illness and my past without having to feel shame or embarrassment anymore. Everything I went through in high school and college was not my fault. I no longer look down on myself.

Sharing my full story has made me wish I didn't go through so many years holding the full weight of my disorder just on myself without asking for help. A lot of my college friends said they would have been more than willing to talk with me about my feelings at that time. They would have supported me. It's made me learn that it's okay to lean on others and ask for help. Mental health is a good thing to talk about! It is way more common to deal with mental health hurdles than you think. Let's normalize talking about it. If I could go back, there would be so many instances where I could have used someone to lean on.

My high school basketball coach, Sellberg, and I reconnected nine years after my senior year and I shared everything with him. He remembers me being down, withdrawn, and moody and that I wasn't acting like myself all season. He told me his biggest frustration was that he could not get me to open up no matter how hard he tried. He didn't know how much to pry and how much to push me without having me shut him out completely. I can't imagine how things would have been different if I had shared with him—a high school health teacher—what I was going through. Reflecting back, it pains me that I tried to do everything alone. I wish I would have asked for help right away and had the correct language to do so.

I no longer identify as Catholic, but I also respect those that choose that as their religion. I don't know if being raised Caltholic and having those rules and rituals enforced within me led to the reason my first psychosis revolved so much around God and the belief of being possessed by a demonic force.

I am a Christian. I have a spiritual relationship with God today and that relationship has helped me grow and given me internal peace. I truly believe in a higher, guiding power. I believe that we are all here to help each other and that is a huge reason why I am sharing my story with you.

Finding True Love

My career was off to a successful start and I was going to counseling with Richard bi-weekly.

In the fall of 2018, I met Ricky Swanson. At this time in my journey I was accepting of my past and more confident than ever. I didn't look down on myself anymore. I reached out to him on social media to ask him if he wanted to go out, and he ended up bringing me on the most awesome first date. We went bowling, grabbed lunch, and attended a Minnesota Vikings game all in the same day. I was immediately swept off my feet and knew he was something special.

Before things got too serious, I told him he needed to know that I had bipolar disorder but was managing it well and was on top of and responsible with my treatment plan. I shared my story with him and told myself if he didn't accept it, I was going to walk away. He gave me a hug, looked lovingly into my eyes, and told me it was okay and he accepted me, all of me. He opened up and told me that he had some family members who dealt with mental health issues, and so he had some understanding and was not scared by it. He even told me I was the least crazy girl he had ever dated. This made me laugh.

October 28th, 2018 journal entry:

> *Today was the most wonderful day. Actually, I had a wonderful weekend. Ricky asked me to be his girlfriend. I have so many feelings for him. I love every second we spend together. He makes me feel beautiful and confident but also a little shy. He accepts all I've been through! I am so overwhelmed by how much I like him. He is cute, funny, takes good care of himself, loves*

> *being active (like me), is affectionate and very*
> *attractive. I love all the time we spend together.*

Our relationship advanced quickly but naturally. Ricky is one of a kind. We share many interests and have a similar outlook on life. He keeps me on my schedule and can call me out if he notices that I'm experiencing any depression or mania.

He is patient and listens to how I am feeling. My life has truly changed for the better since he has come into it. We have so much fun together and he fits in extremely well with my family. We have traveled to so many amazing new places and he shares my appreciation for being active and exploring the outdoors. He's my biggest supporter and also my biggest critic. He pushes me out of my comfort zone and helps me be a better person, and I genuinely love him unconditionally. He is my dream boy.

I truly believe things happen for a reason. If I didn't quit the team, I would have continued to struggle with disordered eating and defining myself by my productivity. If I had not broken up with Joe, I never would have found true love or even known what that felt like. I would not have followed my heart. If I had never re-lived or accepted my experience in Richard's office that one day, and done all the hard work on myself through therapy, I would still be as sad and unsure of who I am and what I am capable of. I would still be living my life in fear. And if I had never had bipolar disorder, I would not have as much empathy for everyone else struggling with mental health hurdles or any health issue for that matter. I would not be the person I am today. I would not have been able to help others through sharing my own story.

January 18th, 2019 journal entry:

> *I am so thankful for all the mistakes in my past because*
> *I've learned from them. I've come to know myself better*
> *and understand what I want in my life. I know I want*
> *Ricky with no doubt in my mind. We have similar*

goals and share a very similar lifestyle. My love for him grows more and more everyday. This is exactly what people mean when they say: "I knew he was the one."

At this point in time, Ricky and I live together and both work from home. I imagine our future kids reading my journals one day. Sometimes I don't want to write down my true feelings in order to shield them from seeing me as in pain or appearing unstable. But that would be doing them an injustice. Life is not always rainbows and butterflies. Everyone struggles with something. Sometimes life is amazing and beautiful and other days it's hard as hell and I want them to see that. I want them to know their mother is strong, confident, and has overcome many obstacles. Someday when they are adults and ready, I will share my journey with them. I will tell them life is far from perfect but it is possible to overcome difficult times. Life is a gift and worth every moment.

Running Free

Sept 19th, 2019 journal entry:

I ran this morning... It's been a while since I laced up my shoes. I did not worry about time or pace, I just ran free and loved every second of it. It made me remember why I've always loved the sport. Now, there is no need for obsessive training, breaking down my body... There is just pure enjoyment and freedom to go however long, short, fast, or slow as my body feels.

Running has taught me so much in life. I've learned to run long, fast, hard and slow. I've learned to win and how to accept a loss. I've learned to push myself more than I ever thought possible. I've learned that comparison steals your joy and that progress takes patience. There is no "special body type" to be a runner. I've learned that walking away from something doesn't necessarily mean quitting, but perhaps taking on something greater. I've learned that life isn't about getting to the end but the relationships and friendships we make along the way. Running is a gift but it does not define me as a person. I am so much more than that.

Accepting Every Season

It was Labor Day weekend in 2020. I was with Ricky and my family at the lake, and we were taking the docks out of the water. It's always a sad time of year because you know fall is on its way. Surprisingly enough, I found I wasn't sad, like so many years past. For the first time I could remember, I was excited for the change in season and what the next chapter had in store.

When I was younger, I would often measure summer by how many dives I would take off of the dock or how many last swims I could make to the rock bar at 9 p.m. and still watch the sunset. I counted because I dreaded time passing and summer fading away. Like it does, time passed and, for a long while, fall meant darker times, mood disruptions, unknown challenges, less time seeing my grandparents, and a faster pace.

Because of my therapist, my self development, my friends and family, and Ricky, I have found inner peace; peace with change of pace, peace with myself and what I've been through. I've accepted that very little of what happens to oneself is in our control, but the way we choose to react and let those experiences affect us is. I believe God brought me to where I was at that moment.

That summer I did not count the swims nor the beautiful sunsets; in fact, I swam less than I ever had. But for some reason I felt more accepting for what was to come and for the colder, shorter days. I wasn't kicking myself for not doing more, running more, experiencing more. I felt at peace and truly happy. I knew as time passed and more things changed, I would always have my memories and I could choose happiness, like Grandpa, even in my darkest times. Summer no longer was the peak of my 365 day cycle. I was free and able to live and choose inner peace always.

My Return to Atlanta

In May of 2021 I went to Florida with Ann and my mom to visit family. Our connecting flight was in the Atlanta airport. I didn't know we would be landing there until I boarded the airplane in Minneapolis. The last time I had been there was when I was eighteen.

As we were flying to Atlanta, I thought about the hospital and all that had transpired there. I thought about how much I despised Georgia. Maybe it didn't have to be that way.

As I walked through the massive airport, I thought about how strange I must have appeared to travelers back in 2013, losing control and being forced to be strapped down. There is a lot I want to understand. *Why did this happen to me the way it did? Why did it have to be so terrifying?* Maybe one day I will know the answer. I thought about how crazy it was that Kylie was there to grab me as I ran past the bathroom. She may have saved my life at that moment. I don't believe that was coincidental.

I thought about how when I have lost touch with reality, I truly lose who I am. It is disturbing to me that I become someone that doesn't represent my true values and respect for myself. I thought about the fact that I truly believed the hallucination and delusions. The brain is so powerful and full of so many unknowns. I never want to lose myself again.

Of course, the airport was only a brief part of my stay here. There is comfort and some good in my memories here.

I remember how awesome my mom was. I remember her coming and seeing me everyday when I didn't think she wanted to see me. I remember the nice nurse, Jen.

I am thankful for all the Reese's Peanut Butter Cups I consumed, how I would savor all of them when my mom would bring them for me. Those Reese's Cups did more than she knew. They were the only thing that tasted good in that hospital. They were chocolatey and sweet and always gave me a brief sense of hope. Whenever I have one today, it makes me smile and think of all the shit I've gotten through. The Reese's taste just as satisfying, but life is so much better and something about that makes me really proud.

I remember talking to Kylie on the phone in the hospital. Even though it was awkward and I wasn't sure what to say, it was comforting to hear her voice. I remember how extremely excited I was to see my dad when he finally came to the hospital to bring me home.

One thing I've got to say about psychiatric hospitals—they really are a place of healing; even the really scary ones. At Cherish, I was forced to get up everyday, eat and take medication. I was forced to live and it allowed me to stabilize. It saved my life. But truly, the real healing comes from within. I would be lying if I said it were easy. I had to accept I wanted to get better and trust others to help me do that.

When you leave a psychiatric hospital, you are in charge again. You have to choose to live a healthy lifestyle. It is your choice what you eat and drink, when and if you take your medication, if you show up to your outpatient psychiatric appointments, if you see a therapist, and who you surround yourself with for support.

Even when I was most depressed, no one was there to tell me to stop sleeping and get out of bed. It takes discipline and hard work and being real with yourself and with those that want to help you. I have done so much work on myself since I was last in Atlanta. I couldn't have done it without the help from my loved ones, my doctor, and therapist. I know for a fact I would not have been able to walk through the airport as confidently and as calmly as I had that day if I had not put in all that hard work and believed in myself.

Managing A Lifelong Journey with Bipolar

Bipolar disorder is a lifelong journey. Even though there is no cure, it is 100 percent treatable and possible to live a fulfilling life. There are so many successful people who have bipolar disorder and you wouldn't even know it. I wish that people would talk about it more. I hope school systems are including it in their curriculum these days to help students.

When I hear stories of a teenager or adult taking their life, I am truly heartbroken because I know how much pain, suffering, and helplessness they felt. It could have been entirely preventable if they had had the help and resources to get them through it. It makes me extremely sad.

Sometimes I go months, even years, without experiencing the familiar symptoms of mania or depression. During these stable periods, I even forget what it feels like and it becomes easy to convince myself there is nothing wrong with me. I tell Richard this and he always tells me, "There was never anything wrong with you." I roll my eyes and try to think of myself in that way.

I know it's common for relapses to happen to people because they decide to stop taking their medication. I never miss a dose of medication or stop taking it even in my most stable times. I remembered what the doctor at Johnson had told me, as long as I was taking medication regularly, I would not lose touch with reality. It is now 2022 and I haven't needed inpatient care for over seven years.

Once in a while I will get caught off guard with a disruption of depression or mania. It takes me a while to realize it, but, after I do, I will go back and look at recent journal entries and see the pattern in my writing as my energy has changed leading up to an episode. Sometimes, Ricky even noticed it before I did.

I am so thankful I don't live alone. Ricky helps to keep me on a schedule. There are days when I struggle to get ready, not oversleep, and do simple tasks such as showering. It is very crucial to me that these barriers do not bleed into how I do my work in my profession or in my relationship with others. Ricky helps me remember what a healthy schedule is.

I am still working to find a clear line between being firm with myself in order to live what I define as a productive and successful life, yet not push myself so far out of my comfort zone that I break. I have goals and expectations for myself to not let this illness define who I am.

Not too long ago, I had a small run in with mania for the first time in over two years. It's not my fault or Ricky's fault, or anyone's fault for that matter; sometimes it just happens.

November 11th, 2021 journal entry:

I can't sleep. I'm wondering if I'm experiencing mania. I am so awake and it's time I should be going to bed. I try so hard to sleep but I feel so much energy pumping through me. I have so many grand ideas for the next canvas I am going to paint. I need to get this energy out. I want to express my inner sensations through art and poetry. But I know it is late and I need to sleep. I've tried meditating and praying, and I just can't get tired. I have a desire to go outside and go on a long walk, but it's late and I know it is unsafe. I feel anxious and uncomfortable laying down. I'm trying really hard to follow my schedule and just breathe. Yesterday I reorganized every cupboard drawer and closet in the entire house. I also labeled most things and made it very neat. A little obsessive, I know...

During this episode I was going to the gym every day and often running outside on my lunch breaks. When I am manic I have a hard time sitting still, am overly productive, spend more money shopping, have an increased sex drive, and obsessively work out. One time I pushed my body during my workout so intensely, because I had so much energy, that I physically injured myself. I've gotten much better with taking care of myself physically and mentally.

But one week later, symptoms of depression started to reappear. A week later I described feelings of depression:

November 17th, 2021 journal entry:

> *Something is off. I had no possible way of making it to the gym today. I'm so exhausted and have no appetite. I took a really long shower and put on comfy clothes. I have a voice in my head telling me to restrict my food. This is just a part of what I deal with. Bad thoughts, mean thoughts; to starve myself and I am unlovable. It is hard to not let the language in my head affect the way I treat myself and view myself. I'm trying to remember that "this too shall pass." I need to continue to live a healthy lifestyle (eat healthy AND enough, take care of my physical health and don't over exercise, meditate, remember what I'm grateful for, lean on Ricky, sleep enough, make an appointment with my psychiatrist). I am so much better than the thoughts in my head. I need to remember the woman I am—the strong, brave, woman I am. Remember who you are. Remember what is important and everything will be okay.*

Even though I've experienced depression many times in my life, it always amazes me that despite the fact that I have come so far and made such positive life changes, depression can still feel like a bitch. It is hollow, painful, dreadful, and tiresome. It is awful beyond words.

I have experienced so many terrible, intrusive thoughts that it doesn't even phase me anymore. I have learned they are just thoughts and they have no power over me. I recognize the thought, tell myself not to listen to it, and use my coping mechanisms to get through it. Just like my moods, they will come and go. I used to think it was a sad thing, to be used to intrusive thoughts; that's not how I look at it anymore. I view it as maturity. I have matured in the way I cope with my illness. I do my best not to fear it.

I never got a clear answer as to why my toxic eating habits always seem to surface when I am unstable. It's like the scenario with the chicken or the egg—which comes first? I don't know if restricting and purging is a result of a mood disruption or if those behaviors are what cause an imbalance. No healthcare professional has been able to give me a clear answer. I do everything I can to not go back to those unhealthy patterns.

When I am struggling with an increase or decrease in mood stability, it is difficult to do the things I need to do to take care of myself.

I do what I can to eat and sleep even when I don't want to. Sometimes it takes leaning on other people to help get me through it. That is the awesome thing about having a supportive network of people I trust. I view my doctors and therapist as my team. I do want to have kids someday, and when I decide it's time, I will have a strong team and support system behind me as well.

Kylie

My relationship with Kylie is stronger than ever. She is still my best friend. We both have a shoe box full of all of the letters we passed back and forth in high school. We both even kept the ones from Johnson.

We have talked about everything from our past in detail, and there is no more pain. I never thought there would be a day where I would sit around a dinner table with both Kylie and Sue and speak so freely about everything that has happened and feel no shame or embarrassment. There was even some laughter. Sue and Kylie are both dear to my heart.

Kylie got her dream job as an occupational therapist and is helping people everyday to improve their quality of life. She even helped me make an emergency care plan in case I ever need to be admitted to the hospital again.

Kylie is always a phone call away if I need a friend to talk to and I'm here for her too. Even though we are both adults with busy schedules, we always make time for each other. We go on walks together at least twice a week in the warmer months and work out together at the gym before work most days as well. Sometimes we even bake together just for old times' sake. We support each other through thick and thin. We truly have been through everything together, and it's only brought us closer. She'll be by my side at my wedding one day, just like we talked about when we were younger. Everyone deserves a friend like Kylie.

Planning for the Future

We can't determine exactly how our future will go, no matter how hard we try. For example, my current job is not what I went to school for, and I would have never imagined myself in the field or role I'm currently in. At one point in my life, I believed I wouldn't have a successful career at all because of my health status. Not only am I maintaining a solid career I enjoy, but I have also been given promotions, new opportunities, and have gained the trust of my team and colleagues to get the job done and get it done well. I have long term goals to continue to advance in the workplace as well.

I would like to continue to break the stigma around mental health injuries and illnesses. I think this is already happening to some degree. I want my story to inspire others and let them know there is hope in recovery. I want to educate more people about bipolar disorder to make sure no one has to go through what I did. I hope to create a world in which teens and adults feel comfortable asking others for help and support. I want to break the stigma which seems to revolve around being diagnosed with bipolar and asking for help.

I also really want kids one day. Some people may think I shouldn't have children. They may think I may be an unstable or unfit mother or that I could possibly pass down mental health issues to my kids. I've thought about all of this in detail, believe me. I don't want to live in fear. I do know I want to be the best mother for my children.

I want to teach my children that it is a good thing to talk about their emotions, and I want Ricky and I to build an environment that feels safe to share good feelings and bad feelings. I want them to know it's okay to ask for help if they ever experience stress or mental health issues.

All the hard work I have done on myself—facing my past, building a treatment plan, having a strong team to stand behind me, believing in myself to live my life with a positive mindset, and choosing happiness everyday—will set me up to be successful in motherhood. I understand I am far from perfect and I do worry about messing up, but that is the case for most new parents in general.

I understand I will need a solid team to support me through the pregnancy process. My OBGYN, psychiatrist, therapist, Ricky, and I will need to work closely together to ensure I am taking care of myself while also growing a healthy baby. I have done plenty of research on my medication and based on conversations with my doctors, we will ensure I am on the safest medication and treatment plan to take care of both the baby and myself.

The future holds so many unknowns, but I do know there will be far more precious and good moments than bad. I am at a point in my life now that I firmly believe I can overcome any and every obstacle, and I will never give up on myself and who I truly am.

How I Define Success

Success for me has changed throughout the years. For a long while, I measured it by how fast I could run, how skinny I was, how productive I could be, what I thought others thought about me.

Some people measure success by how much money they make or what their job title is. Success to me is none of those things. At this point in my life, it is much deeper than that. To laugh often to appreciate the beauty in all seasons; to see the beauty in others; to love fully, fearlessly and be unconditionally loved; to leave the world a bit better and help others along the way; and to live, most days, feeling at peace—peace with who I am, peace with all I've been through, and to feel peace with the unknown and what is yet to come. Success also comes from sharing my story and helping me accept my past.

For roughly four years in my early-mid twenties I experienced recurring dreams almost every night. In my dreams, I was either playing basketball in high school or running down the hallways because I was late for class. In 2022, I got together with my high school principal and Kylie for dinner. We talked about old times and I shared my story with my principal as she was involved in helping me transition back to school in 2013. I shared with her my recurring dreams and she asked me if something was still bothering me about high school. Emotion washed over me and tears streamed down my face. I told her about how hard it was for me to go back to school after going through all that trauma. I shared with her the pain I felt and the way I despised high school because of my depression that I experienced in the classroom, hallways, and on the basketball court. I allowed myself to cry and feel my pain and sadness. After that conversation, I have not had one dream about high school or basketball. It's amazing and beautiful how talking about our experiences can allow us to heal.

Over time, I've put together an art journal, expressing myself through paint, poetry, pictures, stickers, and sketches. I have a drawer filled with almost a dozen journals I've filled over the years. One page is a list of all the things I wish I could tell my younger self.

Things that I Wish I Could Tell my Younger Self:

- ⊙ *You are beautiful inside and out. Your body is amazing. Believe it is perfect just the way God made it and don't try to make it something it's not meant to be. Take care of it because you only get one.*
- ⊙ *Life won't look like you imagined it, it's much better.*
- ⊙ *You are never a burden to anyone. Don't believe any thoughts that tell you otherwise.*
- ⊙ *Just because everyone else is doing something doesn't mean you should too.*
- ⊙ *Moderation is key to everything you do in life.*
- ⊙ *Those terrible things to come, they are not your fault. Release your shame.*
- ⊙ *You won't believe it now, but someday you will meet the man you never knew you needed, and he will help you grow and you will love together.*
- ⊙ *Don't take everything in Catholic Church so literally. Know that God loves you so much, and he is always on your side even when you feel alone.*
- ⊙ *Having your family and health is everything.*
- ⊙ *Open up to your family, friends, coaches, and teachers when you are struggling and having bad thoughts. Share your feelings honestly.*
- ⊙ *Your productivity does not define your worth.*
- ⊙ *Perfectionism is unattainable and chasing it is tiresome. Fall in love with imperfection. Know you are enough.*
- ⊙ *Sometimes there will be pain, but don't be scared and don't give up; for life has more blissful and beautiful moments than the scary ones. Life is worth living.*

National Suicide Hotline # - 800-273-8255 and reach a 24-hour crisis center OR text MHA to 741741

About the Author:

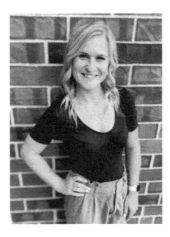

Kate Simonet resides in Minnesota with her boyfriend, Ricky, and their two labradoodles, Teddy and Winnie. When she's not writing or journaling, she can be found traveling or at her family's cabin. This is her first book.

Choosing Happiness, LLC
Instagram: choosing_happiness_llc
Email: *choosing.happiness.llc@gmail.com*

CPSIA information can be obtained
at www.ICGtesting.com
Printed in the USA
LVHW021246210622
721764LV00004B/451